ADVANCE PRAISE FOR *B IS FOR BALANCE: A NURSE'S GUIDE FOR ENJOYING LIFE AT WORK AND AT HOME*

"Sharon Weinstein's *B Is for Balance* helps us connect the dots in the midst of life's chaos and shows us how to access our energy, our vitality, and our calmness each day. This book is a goldmine of easy-to-follow, life-enhancing activities, with how-to's for measuring our balance and finding the time to do it. By following these suggestions and knowledge, we can truly tap into our purpose for living as well as our joy and wisdom."

–Barbara Dossey, PhD, RN, AHN-BC, FAAN
International Co-Director
Nightingale Initiative for Global Health
Author of Holistic Nursing: A Handbook for
Practice (5th ed.); Florence Nightingale Today:
Healing, Leadership, Global Action; and
Florence Nightingale: Mystic, Visionary, Healer

"In today's frenzied world, most of us have more to balance in our lives than ever before. We are driven in a stress-filled, complicated life style that has us wired 24/7. Doing it all, no matter what the cost, is a way of life today. But, we really cannot do it all; we only *think* we can. *B Is for Balance* is a must-read. It makes you focus on responsibility to self and how that will balance your life. Find your balance and let this book help you."

–Rita M. Carty, PhD, RN, FAAN
Professor and Dean Emerita
College of Health and Human Services
George Mason University

"*B Is for Balance* is a truly inspiring book that grabs your attention and makes you stop and think about what's really important in life. I was reminded over and over again how balance can reap astonishing benefits. *B Is for Balance* will undoubtedly compel readers to look inside themselves and examine how they manage competing demands with taking care of themselves. Everyone with a busy life should take time to read this book to rediscover how balance can lead to a more healthy and fulfilled life."

—Colonel John S. Murray, PhD, RN, CPNP, CS, FAAN
President, Federal Nurses Association

"Unlike other books in this genre, *B Is for Balance* addresses the unique concerns of professional nurses who embody the equally important roles of spouse, parent, and friend. The information is timely, relevant, and to the point. Even though this book is a quick read (a real plus for busy professionals), the messages endure well beyond the completion of the final chapter. I immediately found myself wanting to share the gift of this reading with colleagues and family members alike."

—Susan Tocco, MSN, RN, CNS, CNRN, CCNS
Neuroscience Clinical Nurse Specialist
Orlando Regional Medical Center, USA

B IS FOR BALANCE

A nurse's guide for enjoying life at work and at home

Dear [illegible] for your mentorship! Love, [illegible]

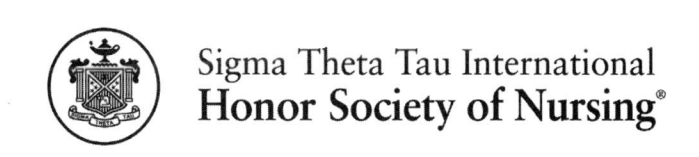

By Sharon M. Weinstein,
MS, RN, CRNI, FAAN

Sigma Theta Tau International
Honor Society of Nursing®

Sigma Theta Tau International

Publisher: Renee Wilmeth
Acquisitions Editor: Cynthia Saver, RN, MS
Development Editor: Carla Hall
Copy Editors: Linda Puffer and Jackie Tirey
Indexer: Angie Bess, RN

Cover Design by: Rebecca Harmon
Interior Design and Page Composition by: Rebecca Harmon

Printed in the United States of America

Sigma Theta Tau International
550 West North Street
Indianapolis, IN 46202

To order additional books, buy in bulk, or order for corporate use, contact Nursing Knowledge International at 888.NKI.4YOU (888.654.4968/U.S. and Canada) or +1.317.634.8171 (outside U.S. and Canada).

To request a review copy for course adoption, send an e-mail to **solutions@nursingknowledge.org,** or contact Cindy Jo Everett directly at 888.NKI.4YOU (888.654.4968/U.S. and Canada) or +1.317.917.4983 (outside U.S. and Canada).

To request author information, or for speaker or other media requests, contact Rachael McLaughlin of the Honor Society of Nursing, Sigma Theta Tau International, at 888.634.7575 (U.S. and Canada) or +1.317.917.4944 (outside U.S. and Canada).

ISBN-13: 978-1-930538-81-8

Library of Congress Cataloging-in-Publication Data

Weinstein, Sharon.
 B is for balance : a nurse's guide for enjoying life at work and at
home / by Sharon M. Weinstein.
    p. ; cm.
 Includes bibliographical references and index.
 ISBN-13: 978-1-930538-81-8
 ISBN-10: 1-930538-81-2
1. Nurses--Life skills guides. I. Title.
 [DNLM: 1. Nurses--psychology. 2. Burnout, Professional--prevention &
control. 3. Nurse's Role--psychology. 4. Quality of Life. 5.
Workload--psychology. WY 87 W424b 2009]
 RT82.W675 2009
 610.73--dc22
                            2009000909

First Printing
2009

DEDICATION

A mom, wife, educator, clinician, international consultant …
I lived a life that others dream about, and all of the pieces
seemed to fit. It was becoming a grandmother that opened
my eyes to a life in balance and what it could do for me and
others!

To my grandchildren—for creating a level of awareness in
me that I have come to love and enjoy, each and every day!

SMW

ACKNOWLEDGEMENTS

In today's health care environment, nurses find themselves pulled in many directions. Nursing has become a balancing act, and we need to stop, for just a few moments, and rethink the need for balance in our lives. How can nurses care for others when they have no time to care for themselves? How can nurses continue to be the best they can possibly be to family, patients, employer, and themselves? This book is about you, the nurse from any walk of life. This book is about the countless number of professionals who walk the walk and talk the talk—toward a balanced life.

I transitioned toward a balanced life with support from my nurse colleagues, mentors, and friends. I transitioned toward a balanced life through the love of my family. Like a house, a balanced lifestyle must have a good foundation. My foundation is firmly rooted; it has evolved from many who have touched my life in many ways:

To my husband, Steve, who taught me to dream big dreams.

To members of my family, for their constant belief in me and in my ability to be all things to all people!

A special thank you to the team of professionals from Sigma Theta Tau International, including Cindy Saver, acquisitions editor; Carla Hall, development editor; and the talented team of copy editors, Linda Puffer and Jackie Tirey. Thanks to Angie Bess, for expert indexing of the manuscript. As we considered a book cover that would reflect the concept of *B Is for Balance,* Rebecca Harmon came to the rescue with a cover design that truly depicts the concept of achieving balance in one's life at home and at work. Thank you, Rebecca, for a terrific design. And, finally, thanks to the contributing authors—

each has found balance in her life and is willing to share it with our reading audience. These are lessons learned, from those who have lived them.

ABOUT THE AUTHORS

Led by Sharon Weinstein, the author team combines the talents and wellness perspectives of five seasoned leaders with powerful backgrounds in practice, process, holistic health, and education.

SHARON M. WEINSTEIN, MS, RN, CRNI, FAAN

President and founder of Core Consulting Group and Core Wellness International, Sharon is the author of six texts and more than 150 peer-reviewed publications. Recent publications include *Nursing Without Borders: Values, Wisdom, and Success Markers*, co-edited with Ann Marie T. Brooks; *Plumer's Principles and Practice of Intravenous Therapy*, eighth edition; and chapters in *Core Curriculum for Infusion Nursing,* fourth edition, and *Educating Nurses for Leadership*. A member of the Medical Wellness Association, Infinity Foundation, Chicago Healers, American Wellness Institute, and American Holistic Nurses Association, Sharon has been seen on NBC 5 Chicago and other media outlets on topics such as attitude, balance, water for health, safe schools, and more. She is the founder of the Integrative Health Forum (IHF), an interdisciplinary alliance of licensed health care professionals whose mission is to serve the professionals and associations that promote health and well-being in individuals, organizations, and communities around the globe (www.ihfglobal.com).

A former member of the Sigma Theta Tau International Leadership Succession Committee, Sharon served as a member of the Governance Council and is a member of Alpha Lambda Chapter. She is a fellow of the American Academy of Nursing and a member of the academy's Expert Panel on Global Nursing. She earned a master's degree in health management and gerontology from North Texas State University, a certificate in health administration from Trinity University, a bachelor's degree in nursing and behavioral science from Wilmington College, and a diploma from Pennsylvania Hospital School of Nursing. She is a graduate of the Kellogg School of Management's Executive Management Program. She is adjunct clinical assistant professor at the University of Illinois at Chicago College of Nursing.

DEBBIE REYNOLDS HUGHES, MSN, APRN, BC, NP-C

Debbie, a dually certified nurse practitioner in family medical and psychiatric mental health, offers patients a holistic approach to health care. In this capacity, she works with clients interested in health promotion, preventive aging medicine, and bio-identical hormone replacement therapy. Her expertise in medical and mental health provides holistic care and thorough evaluation and treatment of symptoms. She worked for 20 years in west-central Nebraska as a registered nurse in a variety of medical settings, including hospital medical/surgical units, home and community health, public schools, and long-term care. In 2002, Debbie moved to Lincoln, Nebraska, where she established her practice after earning a Master of Science in Nursing degree from the University of Nebraska. In 2006, she founded Holistic Harmony Inc., a corporation committed to providing holistic comprehensive care and wellness. She is certified as a psychiatric/mental health nurse practitioner with the American Academy of Nurse Practitioners and as a family nurse practitioner with the American Nurses Credentialing Center. She is a member of the Nebraska Nurses Association, Nebraska Nurse Practitioners, American Academy of Nurse Practitioners, and American Holistic Nurses Association.

HOLLY TIMBERLAKE, PHD

Holly took a giant leap in 2003 from holistic psychologist (one who assists others in healing from emotional wounds by attending also to the physical and spiritual aspects of a person) to holistic businesswoman, life coach, and cultural creative nurturer. Many influences came together to create Nakaia Healing Arts, including her passions for spiritual development and community building, and her beliefs in the possibilities of radiant and vibrant living, healing, and growth. A writer and public speaker, she conducts retreats and facilitates workshops. Holly is passionate about family and friends, the outdoors, beauty, writing, dancing and singing, and unleashing her own creativity in the world. She has just finished an ebook called *Joyously Green: Holiday Living and Giving* and is beginning a blog of the same name and a daily enewsletter of guided Emotional Freedom Technique (EFT) sessions. Her Web site is www.nakaia.com, and her e-mail address is hollyt@nakaia.copm.

MADELINE R. ZAWORSKI, MSN, MBA, RN, FACHE, CNAA

A certified wellness consultant, Madeline is owner of A Time for Balance-Wellness in the greater Cleveland area. She holds an executive MBA from Weatherhead School of Management and an MSN from Frances Payne Bolton School of Nursing, Case Western Reserve University. She is a J&J Wharton Nurse Executive Fellow and a fellow of the American College of Healthcare Executives. Madeline is an accomplished health care professional with experience in acute care environments and academia. She has made a successful transition as a wellness entrepreneur in alternative practice and is actively involved in health, wellness, and civic leadership. A founding member of the Integrative Health Forum, Madeline is a frequent presenter at wellness programs.

DONNA BYRNE, BSCN, MSCN

Donna earned both her Bachelor of Science in Nursing and her Master of Science in Nursing from McGill University. The owner/director of Health Access Community Care, she has been a health care professional for more than 30 years. Both as a staff nurse and a nursing administrator, Donna has served the Montreal, Quebec, communities, developing services to meet varying and changing health care needs. She created Health Access Community Care, which is dedicated to health promotion and prevention through assisting individuals and their families in remaining healthy and as independent as possible. By using a combination of traditional health care, learning, and alternative approaches, Health Access staff members promote achievement of optimum health and wellness within the community. Committed to health learning, Donna has hosted a radio show called "The Wellness Plan." She most recently developed a Télésanté (French translation for e-health) program for home care to help individuals stay in their homes safely. The Sante-TELE-Health research program began in early 2008 with a McGill University colleague, Dr. Antonia Arnaert. A 3-month COPD trial has been completed, and a hypertension study using Blackberry technology has been initiated.

TABLE OF CONTENTS

INTRODUCTION

What is this thing called balance? You hear about it everywhere, you read about it, and you long for it. But what *is* it? What does it look like? And, is it possible for normal people with jobs, families, hobbies, and multiple internal and external commitments to achieve balance in our modern world? The last answer is, of course, a resounding *yes*!

For most people, a balanced life means having optimal time to give to their families, their work, their communities, and their extracurricular and spiritual activities. It also means having enough money or compensation to meet all the basic needs of existence and to save for future needs and desires. For most people, work consumes the majority of their day, and they have to fit family, shopping for and preparing food, and extracurricular activities as they can into their remaining time. Diet and optimal sleep frequently suffer when people are trying to do everything they need or want to do in a limited amount of "free" time. Relationships also suffer.

Nurses and other health care professionals know about balance and are the first to encourage their patients and clients to find balance in their lives. Unfortunately, nurses and health care professionals frequently find themselves doing the opposite of what they recommend: They work too much, they don't eat well, they sleep too little, they don't exercise, and they don't slow down when they get sick. There's always too much to do—at home, at work, at the kids' schools—for our training and education endeavors, and for our personal and professional goals.

While it seems a daunting task to slow down enough to consider and contemplate achieving balance, it is a task worth doing—one that will improve your life in expected ways, but also in ways that may come to surprise you.

BENEFITS OF ACHIEVING BALANCE

Achieving balance in your life can bring you amazing rewards. You can expect some or all of the following changes and improvements in your life as you move into balance:

- Improved health, including lower blood pressure and cholesterol levels
- Less stress and more happiness
- More energy
- Improved quality of life
- Better relationships
- Improved concentration
- More free time
- Potentially longer lifespan
- Sustainable health
- Simplicity in your life

HOW THIS BOOK CAN HELP YOU ACHIEVE BALANCE

This book was written to help nurses and health care professionals learn how to balance their work and home lives. It is an active book. While we give you sufficient information, anecdotes, and wisdom to inform your work, the goal is to move you into balance. Some of the features to help you achieve that goal are:

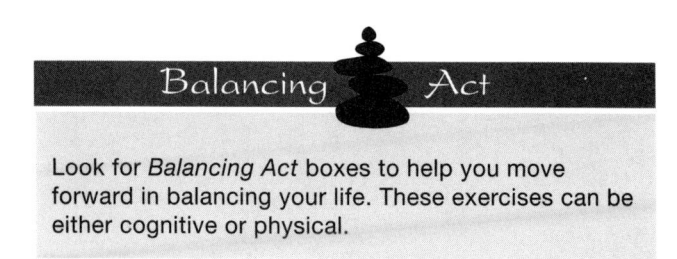

Balancing Act

Look for *Balancing Act* boxes to help you move forward in balancing your life. These exercises can be either cognitive or physical.

Keeping Your Balance

Keeping Your Balance boxes are at the end of each chapter. These exercises reinforce the message of the chapter and support your move toward a balanced life.

RESOURCES

You will find resources and further readings at the end of each chapter to help you explore specific topics in more detail.

RECOVERING YOUR BALANCE

The challenge for all of us is to truly create balance in our lives, given the limitations of time and money. It is a significant commitment to take the first steps toward recovering your balance in life, but those steps will reward you and your family many times over the actual investment.

Balance is an ideal, to be sure, and while you cannot use a PDA to program balance into your life, it is within reach. The exercises in this chapter are not difficult. The difficulty lies in the commitment it takes to retake control of your life. Read on and begin the journey toward your own personal balance.

PART I
Balancing Without Acting

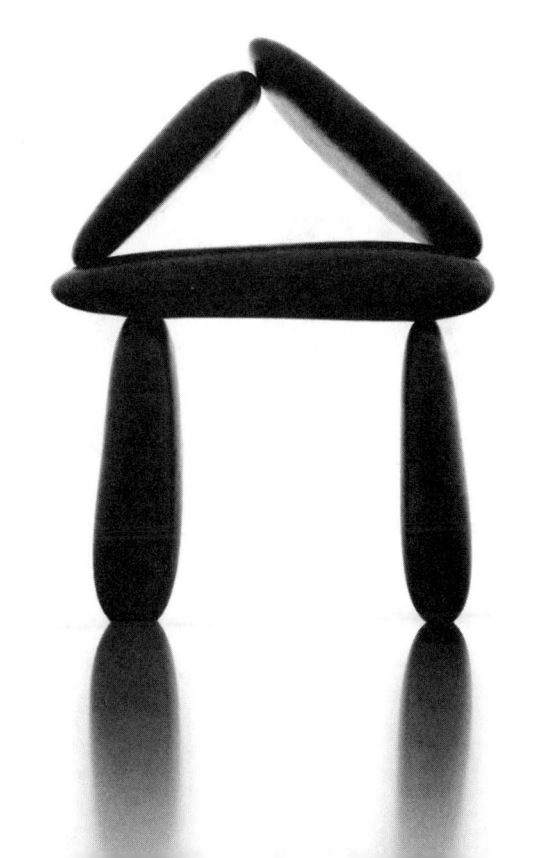

"Many men go fishing all of their lives without knowing it is not fish they are after."

—Henry David Thoreau

1

KNOWING YOUR PURPOSE

We all want to believe our lives are meaningful and that at the end of our lives, we will have had a positive impact on the world. We seek meaning—physically, emotionally, and spiritually—through our work, our families, and our communities. Many nurses go into their profession because they want their everyday work to have meaning. Unfortunately, like all humans, nurses can find themselves lost and purposeless, and their lives unfulfilling.

WHY AM I HERE?

Life purpose is not simply our work lives, nor is it simply our home lives or our roles within our families and communities. It is a combination—a balance, if you will—of all aspects of our lives that creates fulfillment. Life purpose is what gives meaning to our lives. It makes us feel alive, empowered, capable, and strong. Life purpose answers the question "Why am I here?"

"Life is not the way it's supposed to be. It's the way it is. The way you deal with it is what makes the difference."

—Virginia Satir

The fortunate among us discover their life purpose. You, too, can be one of those fortunate ones. This chapter presents clear and simple ways for you to identify your life's purpose and to prepare yourself for living out that purpose.

WHY IDENTIFY YOUR LIFE PURPOSE?

1. It gives meaning to everything you do.
2. It directs and guides you.
3. It motivates you.

You are reading this book, and that means you are looking to achieve balance in your life. To find that balance, you must first know where your center is. Finding your purpose will give you that center necessary for achieving balance. It's an important task, and one that should not be skipped. You cannot read about it, listen to someone telling you what to do, or do anything other than discover the purpose of your life on your own.

Ask yourself . . . What gives your life meaning?

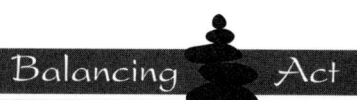

Balancing Act

A SIMPLE APPROACH TO FINDING YOUR LIFE PURPOSE

If you want to discover your true purpose in life, you must first empty your mind of all the false purposes you've been taught (including the idea that you may have no purpose at all).

So, how do you discover your purpose in life? While there are many ways to do this, some of them fairly involved, here is one of the simplest that anyone can do. The more open you are to this process, and the more you expect it to work, the faster it will work for you. Being closed to it, having doubts about it, or thinking it's a meaningless exercise won't prevent it from working as long as you stick with it. It will just take longer to converge.

HERE'S WHAT TO DO:

Take out a blank sheet of paper or log onto your computer and open a blank document. I prefer the latter because it's faster, but writing manually helps some. Choose the approach that will help you persist in the exercise.

- Write at the top, "What is my true purpose in life?"

- Write an answer (any answer) that pops into your head. It doesn't have to be a complete sentence. A short phrase is fine.

- Repeat the step above until you write the answer that makes you cry. This is your purpose.

That's it. It doesn't matter if you're a nurse, counselor, engineer, or bodybuilder. To some people, this exercise will make perfect sense. To others it will seem ridiculous. It should take about 15-20 minutes to clear your head of all the clutter and the social conditioning about what you think your purpose in life is. The false answers will come from your mind and your memories. But when the true answer finally arrives, it will feel like it's coming to you from a different source entirely.

For those who are entrenched in low-awareness living, it will take a lot longer to get all the false answers out, possibly more than an hour. But if you persist, after 100 or 200 or maybe even 500 answers, you'll be struck by the answer that causes you to surge with emotion, the answer that breaks you. If you've never done this, it may very well sound silly to you. So let it seem silly, and do it anyway.

As you go through this process, some of your answers will be similar. You may even re-list previous answers. Then you might head off on a new tangent and generate 10-20 more answers along some other theme. And that's fine. You can list whatever answer pops into your head as long as you just keep writing.

At some point during the process (typically after about 50-100 answers), you may want to quit and just can't see it converging. You may feel the urge to get up and make an excuse to do something else. That's normal. Push past this resistance, and just keep writing. The feeling of resistance will eventually pass.

You may also discover a few answers that give you a mini-surge of emotion, but they don't quite make you cry—they're just a bit off. Highlight those answers as you go along, so you can come back to them to generate new permutations. Each reflects a piece of your purpose, but individually is not complete. When you start getting these kinds of answers, it just means you're getting warm. Keep going.

It's important to do this alone and with no interruptions. If you're a nihilist, then feel free to start with the answer, "I don't have a purpose," or "Life is meaningless," and take it from there. If you keep at it, you'll still eventually converge.

When I did this exercise, it took me about 30 minutes and 93 steps to reach my final answer. Partial pieces of the answer (mini-surges) appeared throughout the process. When I felt resistance midstream, I took a break,

closed my eyes, meditated, ;
was helpful, as the answers I
began to have greater clarity.

My final answer was: to live c
geously; to resonate with love
awaken the great spirits within
lives in the process; and to lea

When you find your own unique
tion of why you're here, you will ......resonate with you
deeply. The words will seem to have a special energy
to you, and you will feel that energy whenever you read
them.

Discovering your purpose is the easy part. The hard part
is keeping it with you on a daily basis and working on
yourself to the point where you become that purpose. I
carry my copy with me wherever I go and repeat it daily.

If you're inclined to question why and how the process
works, wait until you have completed it yourself. Once
you've done that, you'll probably have your own answer
as to why it works. And, if you ask 10 different people
why this works (people who've successfully completed
it), you'll get 10 different answers, all filtered through
their individual belief systems, and each will contain its
own reflection of truth.

Obviously, this process won't work if you quit before
convergence. I'd guesstimate that 80-90% of people
should achieve convergence in less than an hour. If
you're really entrenched in your beliefs and resistant to
the process, maybe it will take you five sessions and 3
hours, but I suspect that such people will simply quit
within the first 15 minutes or won't attempt it at all. But
if you're drawn to the process, you will finish it. Give it a
shot! You have everything to gain, and nothing at all to
lose.

urself . . . What do you notice as the
n themes in your life?

SELF-KNOWLEDGE

Once you've identified your life's purpose, or are working hard
on it, learning more about yourself—your habits, strengths,
and weaknesses—is important for the next steps. If you have
true friends, you have an important source of self-knowledge.
Real friends will tell you the truth about yourself, and they
don't need to be asked to do so. Keep your friends close
while you are identifying your life purpose and seeking self-
knowledge. Share with them your explorations, and ask for
their input and support. Reflect on their knowledge of your
habits, strengths, and weaknesses. If it feels safer, establish
ground rules so you do not feel attacked. Seek input only from
friends whom you trust completely.

The following section explores other means of self-
knowledge, focusing on seeking out influential people and
trusting intuition.

INFLUENTIAL PEOPLE

Influential people are leaders who have vision, courage, persistence, confidence, generosity, integrity, creativity, enthusiasm,
character, and virtue. They have the ability to retain these
qualities in the midst of chaos, confusion, and difficulty. They
are extraordinary, and their presence energizes and inspires
people. They rarely criticize anything or anyone, because they
are too busy fulfilling their purpose and getting the job done.

They can be a grandparent, parent, friend, business contact, professional colleague, supervisor, or complete stranger.

Identifying influential people is important, because we can learn and grow from their strength of character and purpose. Victor Frankl has been influential in the lives of many. From Frankl's experiences in concentration camps during World War II, including Auschwitz and Dachau, he observed that life has meaning under all conditions, and that it is psychologically damaging when a person's meaning in life is blocked. In his 1997 book, *Man's Search for Meaning*, he wrote that it is possible to find meaning in suffering.

"Fundamentally, therefore, any man can, even under such circumstances, decide what shall become of him—mentally and spiritually. He may retain his human dignity even in a concentration camp."

—Victor Frankl

Frankl's recommendation was to let life question you. What he meant is that life questions us through circumstances such as terminal disease, divorce, and the death of loved ones. He believed that we benefit from crises in that we are forced to let go of petty concerns, conflicts, and the need for control. Even smaller crises can inform our days and our purpose. What did that near-miss car accident at the intersection this morning tell you? Were you rushing? Not paying attention? How would the difference of a few seconds one way or the other have changed your day or your life—short- or long-term? What about that new patient down the hall who makes you think of someone in your life, past or present? How do the thoughts or questions arising from that contact bring new or different meaning to your life?

Seek out influential people whose work speaks to your core beliefs and life purpose. Study their lives and their choices, and take strength from their struggles to fulfill their life work. Go back in history or go forward. Even children can be role models, reminding us of what really matters in life.

Work to emulate the person who influences and inspires you, and develop those qualities and behaviors that you recognize as important. Be a leader and do not be afraid to show your authentic self. Dare to live the life most people only dream about. Think of Albert Einstein's words when you meet criticism: "Great spirits have always encountered violent opposition from mediocre minds."

Ask yourself . . . What is your contribution meant to be during your lifetime?

INTUITION AND SELF-AWARENESS

To discover our purpose, we must trust our intuition. The key to acting *on purpose* is to bring together the needs of the world with our unique gifts and talents. Working on purpose gives us a sense of direction. Life purpose comes from within and expresses itself in almost every aspect of life. The more we are in touch with our life purpose, the more we will notice how it drives us as an internal motivating factor to achieve what we want.

Purpose depends on intuition. Intuition is the inner voice that leads to purpose. It is a sixth sense. It is independent of conscious reasoning. Sometimes, we cannot explain how we "know" something; we just do. Most people know how to get what they *think* they want, but many do not know *what* they want.

To heighten your intuitiveness, you must first be aware of your needs. Psychologist Abraham Maslow (1943) arranged the array of fundamental human needs into a hierarchy. The most basic are physiological needs and safety. First, he argued, we must meet our physiological needs—oxygen, nutrition, and sleep—and feel secure that we are safe. The next level is emotion—love and affection. Next, Maslow concluded, even if physical, safety, and emotional needs are met, discontentment and restlessness will soon develop unless we are doing what we are passionate about—in other words, unless we are fulfilling our higher needs or purpose. Finally, to feel ultimate peace, we must listen to our inner calling, or what Maslow referred to as self-actualization. At this highest level, we live with purpose. This is the level at which those who seek to emulate lives of service—modeled on Nightingale, Gandhi, Mandela, and Mother Theresa—operate so effectively.

Psychologist Clayton Alderfer (1972) compressed Maslow's levels into three, known as the ERG Theory:

1. Existence
2. Relatedness
3. Growth

Alderfer's theory is less rigid than Maslow's. According to ERG, needs can be pursued simultaneously and in any order.

People who can't meet their growth needs will revert to other needs, he argues.

When considering your needs, remember that everything in life is a choice. We choose the food we eat, the clothes we wear, and most importantly, we choose the thoughts we think. We are moving toward our purpose from birth to death and are forced to make choices along the way. This is life's greatest truth and most difficult lesson. Choices give us the power to be ourselves and live the life we have imagined. As we develop our intuitiveness, we will grow in the self-awareness that we are living the life of our choices up to this point, and we have the freedom to change our lives going forward.

DEFINE WHO YOU WANT TO BE

Being *on purpose* means living your life intentionally, with purpose to all your actions. The meaning and purpose of your life is for you to become the best person you can be. When we discover ourselves and who that best person is that we want to become, everything begins to make sense to us. Until we discover our essential purpose, little makes sense.

"Don't be afraid your life will end; be afraid that it will never begin."

—Grace Hansen

What do you want in life? Do you seek the things that money can buy or the things that money cannot buy? If you had to rank the following in order, how would you rank them?

- Possessions
- Personal relationships
- Professional success

People today are more distracted and busier than at any point in history. We have more material possessions and are highly interconnected through our social activities, but too often something is still missing. Many people perceive their purpose in relation to success in the workplace and financial independence. For example, many allow themselves to be part of a society of people rushing around and working too much, just so they can indulge themselves in material possessions. Most of us want to put (or say that we *do* put) our personal relationships first, but in what way? Do we spend time with our friends and loved ones in deep, intimate conversation about ourselves, our relationships, our purpose, and how to live out our days with intention? Or, do we spend time with them running here and there—to the mall, to the movies, to the next commitment in a long list of commitments? Our sound-bite conversations may come close to intimacy—"sharing" about spouses, our weight, a health care issue, or a family concern—but then we're interrupted and the moment is lost.

Think about your life. Is it all caught up in rushing and consuming? What do you want it to be about? Can you visualize your life as you want it to be?

SETTING GOALS

A goal is the next step after discovering our purpose and what we want to achieve in the course of our lives. A goal must first be specific and measurable. Think of a goal as a dream with expectations. It is not a goal if we cannot define it fully nor determine whether we achieved it.

Set goals that will stretch you to the limits but not over-whelm you. These are called "stretch goals." They must be sufficiently difficult, but not impossible. Remember that goal setting is important in developing our level of hope. Positive psychologists who study hope are clear that hope consists not only of willpower, but also meaningful goals to which we apply our will.

"If you do nothing unexpected, nothing unexpected happens."

—Fay Weldon

Start by setting goals to give you small victories that build your confidence in every area of your life. If you don't know what you want from life, everything will appear either as an obstacle or as a burden. One of the great lessons is that the whole world gets out of the way for people who know what they want or where they are going. Be assured—if you do not know where you are going, you are lost. You are never too young or too old to do what you want in life.

Tiger Woods was 3 years old when he shot 48 for nine holes on his hometown golf course. Mozart was 8 years old when he wrote his first symphony. Bill Gates was 19 years old when he co-founded Microsoft. Susan B. Anthony was 49 when she co-founded the National Women's Suffrage Association that eventually led to women's rights in the United States. Michelangelo was 72 when he designed the dome of St. Peter's Basilica in Rome. No matter your age, you can change your destiny.

There are moments when you might feel confused about your purpose in life. Living with the following core beliefs will make your destiny much clearer.

- Believe that your beliefs and attitudes structure how the world appears and that your intuition is guiding you to fulfill your purpose.

- Honestly admit what is working in your life and what is not, and commit only to those things that have heart and meaning for you.

- Keep your life simple. You will attract people and events at the appropriate time, so stop struggling for power and control.

Above all, remember that you always have a choice.

To stay focused on your purpose in all areas of your life, here are some suggestions:

- Control your physical cravings, and do not be a slave to food, drink, or any other substance.

- Identify the people, activities, and possessions that are most important to you, and give them your precious time.

- Cultivate the courage, determination, and persistence to choose the path you are passionate about following, and serve others in the process.

- Share your wealth with all you can, and by doing so you will grow in personal wealth and never again be in need.

- Find true love with a soul mate who challenges and cherishes you.

- Maintain a sense of peace in knowing who you are.

ALIGNMENT WITH PURPOSE

The 21st century challenges us with a new global economy and technology-driven world that is changing rapidly. Thomas Friedman (2005) calls it a "flat world" in that the playing field is level, and individuals from around the planet can connect, communicate, and compete for our planet's limited resources. We are closing out the final chapters of the Industrial Age and opening up a new chapter that many believe is the "spiritual age." This spiritual age is not defined in a religious sense, but more broadly reflects the belief that the search for meaning and living a life of values and purpose is what is most important.

We can easily recognize those, including ourselves, who are aligned with their purpose. The world is full of people who work too much, sleep too little, lead a sedentary lifestyle, eat food that lacks nutritional value, and never have enough time to spend with friends and family. We need to refocus, because our lifestyles are destroying our well-being.

Why is it so important to be aligned with our purpose? Because when we are *on purpose*, we have more energy and true happiness in our lives. Being in alignment with our purpose gives us peace. Peace is not the absence of pain. Peace is a certainty of living life for a worthy purpose, knowing that we are becoming a better person and touching the lives of others every day.

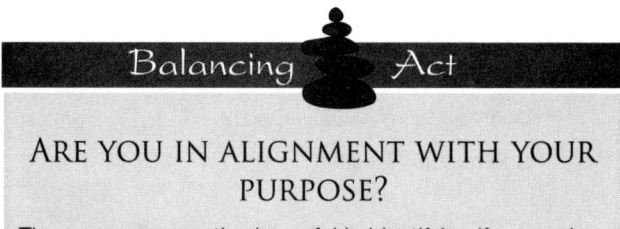

ARE YOU IN ALIGNMENT WITH YOUR PURPOSE?

There are many methods useful in identifying if we are in alignment with our purpose. For example, we may ask ourselves, "Do I wake up most days feeling energized to go to work?" If the answer is "yes," then we may have an indication of our degree of alignment. Other questions to ask ourselves include "Do my talents add real value to people's lives?" and "Can I be my authentic self at work?" At the end of the day, do we feel satisfied about how our day was spent? And when we are at home and with our families and friends, do we feel at peace and content?

It is important to align ourselves with our purpose by prioritizing what is important to us. If we fail to do this, we are sacrificing our holistic health—physically, emotionally, intellectually, and spiritually. We must decide what is really important and necessary and make time for it. Otherwise, life will keep us distracted from what is really important. When we are attentive to our legitimate needs, we will find peace and fulfillment.

Your life is a vast array of choices that can bring you closer to the person you want to become. Bring into your life whatever you desire by deciding who you are and what you need to be happy. As Henry David Thoreau said, "If one advances confidently in the direction of one's dreams, and endeavors to live the life which one has imagined, one will meet with a success unexpected in common hours." Are you pursuing your dreams?

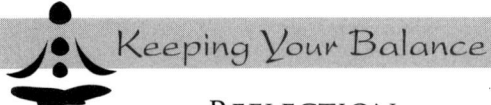 Keeping Your Balance

REFLECTION

- Who are the influential people in your life? What are their qualities?

- Do I have a sense of purpose?

- Do I trust my intuition?

CREATE AN ELEVATOR SPEECH

Here is an exercise to help define your purpose. It sounds simple, but it is a very challenging exercise. Develop an "elevator pitch." Identify your life's purpose and learn to state it as if in conversation. If you can state your life's purpose with another person in the time it takes to ride an elevator—approximately 60 seconds—then you have clarity around your life purpose.

GOAL SETTING

Create a goal that is SMART:

- Specific

- Measureable

- Achievable

- Realistic

- Timely

Example: You never eat vegetables but want to start. Don't expect to go from none to five a day. Instead, create a more realistic goal such as: Beginning on Monday, I'll eat two servings of vegetables each day. I'll keep track of when I eat a vegetable by marking it on the calendar.

Let's say you eat two servings of vegetables a day for the next 3 weeks. Then revise your goal upward to three servings of vegetables, etc.

"Poverty is involuntary and debilitating, whereas simplicity is voluntary and enabling."

—Duane Elgin

2

SIMPLIFY YOUR LIFE

Maintaining a work/life balance is essential for our well-being. The best way to begin working toward that balance is to simplify your life. Keeping it simple is a voluntary process, and you have the power to achieve this goal.

Nursing has always been a challenging endeavor. The origins of nursing as we know it today are often traced to the Crimean War experiences of Florence Nightingale and others associated with the British Army. While much has been written about the work of Nightingale serving the troops, she is best known for her contribution to the decrease in morbidity and mortality of wounded soldiers through the application of basic statistical analysis, infection control measures, and what we now call quality improvement procedures.

From the early days of Nightingale serving the troops to nursing's current milieu, nurses have worked long hours in trying circumstances to serve those in their care. As nurses, we find gratification in serving others, but in the process, our own needs are frequently neglected. Each of us, at one time or another, has felt overwhelmed. We hesitate to take a holiday because when we return, the paperwork will be piled sky-high. We hesitate to attend a professional development program for fear of the seemingly insurmountable volume of work that awaits our return.

A COMPLEXITY EXIT

The sheer complexity of our lives creates internal distress and can wreak havoc on our bodies. Distress is a contributor to disease. The cardiac system is over-stimulated, the immune system is suppressed, and our hormones are out of balance. The complex endocrine system controls the way you respond to your surroundings and provides the proper amount of energy your body needs to function. Hormone imbalances result in a multitude of diseases, including, but not limited to, diabetes, osteoporosis, pituitary disorders, and thyroid conditions. While some are more serious than others, these conditions have debilitating effects on physical and emotional health and quality of life for increasing numbers of professionals.

"The ability to simplify means to eliminate the unnecessary so that the necessary may speak."

—Hans Hofmann

Complexity is addictive, and we cannot always find a way out. I know, because I've been there. When I was first introduced to the concept of work/life balance in 2002, I realized that I needed to radically change my own life. I understood that simplification could have a very positive impact on my work, my family, and my health—and I set out on a mission to simplify my own life. For me, this required a huge paradigm shift, and likely will for you, too.

Balancing Act

BEGINNINGS: MY JOURNEY TO SIMPLICITY

My life is simplified now, compared to the years between 1992 and 2004, when I worked about 100 hours per week and traveled monthly to countries in Eastern Europe. At that time, I directed the office of international affairs for a large hospital alliance, and 50% of my time was subcontracted to the United States Agency for International Development (USAID). My role was to foster international partnerships between U.S. hospitals and their foreign counterparts. I loved the work, I loved the people with whom I interacted, and I loved my job. The hours were extreme, and I found myself in a constant state of catching up and was always tired. Now, with a self-imposed work week of 40 hours, I feel I have dramatically simplified my life. I now have time to work, write, teach, be with family, and give back to society.

I've taken lessons learned in less-developed countries to heart as I have simplified my life. In my travels, I witnessed firsthand how simple life can be. Immediately following the earthquake in Yerevan, Armenia, on December 7, 1988, the only decent housing was in a former government hotel. Although we had neither heat nor hot water, I had a roof over my head and a clean bed. When there was no food in the hospital, our hosts found moldy bread. We ate this for weeks—sometimes with cheese or tomato sauce—and always with an appreciation for what we had. Although it was impossible to get hot water in a tub, we could use an electric coil to warm some water and rinse the shampoo out of our hair. Our colleagues lacked so much, but their refinement of spirit and passion for their work were unsurpassed. They lived a simple life—nearly a sparse life—yet a life of gratitude.

A PERSONAL CHOICE

Simplifying one's life is a personal choice as well as a process. To start, examine your life and determine at least five areas that can be simplified (*see* sidebar, Simplify by Five). While you may be habituated to taking care of all the laundry or dishes, can you release yourself from perfectionism and teach the kids or spouse how to do it? Even though it may take some restraint to keep from judging their efforts, identify the rewards for each of you if you successfully transition a task or responsibility to someone else in the household. What about the evening or morning routines? Look closely at everything you do to identify those five complicated parts of your life that can be simplified.

"Any intelligent fool can make things bigger, more complex, and more violent. It takes a touch of genius—and a lot of courage—to move in the opposite direction."

—E.F. Schumacker

I had the unfortunate experience of having my home for sale for more than a year. Because of this, we had to always be ready for an impromptu realtor visit with prospective buyers. Each and every day we had to make the beds, fill the dishwasher, put away the laundry, and clean the countertops. Because we had educated ourselves on all the "tips" for piquing a buyer's interest, we kept fresh flowers in the kitchen and bathrooms and maintained an uncluttered environment. We had to do all this with already complicated schedules. To help myself out, I had floral arrangements created to mimic fresh ones so that these could be placed at a moment's notice. While I would have preferred fresh flowers, I helped reduce the stress in my already stressful life by eliminating that small task.

Balancing Act

SIMPLIFY BY FIVE

Think of five areas in your life and begin your process to simplify. Write down each area. These areas could be work, food/nutrition, exercise, family, school, community, professional affiliations, and extracurricular activities.

Some Solutions

- Would your work go smoother if you spent a little time before work organizing? Look at everything you do on a daily basis and determine areas where you could be more efficient or eliminate duplication. Propose changes to make yourself, your work, your area more efficient.

- Eat foods prepared simply, but eat with family and friends, or make a ritual out of it, with each person being responsible for one aspect of the meal. Even school-age kids can be responsible for putting together a salad, fresh vegetable dish (or steamed vegetable with help from adults), and simple grains, and parents can trade off on the main course preparation. Everyone can work together before the beginning of the week to create a menu and a meal plan, and do the shopping.

- Look at your community or professional affiliation responsibilities. Drop membership on a committee to free your time.

- Create a community with other parents to trade off carpooling to and from sports practice, drama club, Scouts, the library, and so on.

- Clear out the clutter in your life to make it easier to find what you need. One solution is to process paperwork by handling it only once. Take action immediately on those items that require only a simple response. Create a system for managing follow-up items, whether a simple "tickler" file or by using a manual or electronic calendar. Put things in their place so that you can find them again.

- Do the laundry every other day and straighten up—but do not clean—every day.

- Turn on the TV only when you have a program to watch.

Other simplification strategies and techniques include meditation, primordial sound meditation, and quantum leaps.

MEDITATION

"You must learn to be still in the midst of activity and to be vibrantly alive in repose."
                                                    —Indira Gandhi

Meditation benefits the mind, body, and spirit. Through inner exploration, meditation awakens our creativity, promotes healing, and transforms us. During meditation, we explore our essential nature, restoring the memory of wholeness in our lives, and we discover pure awareness. It begins with concentration—trying to focus your mind on any one point. Meditation is broadly classified under the term "mind-body medicine."

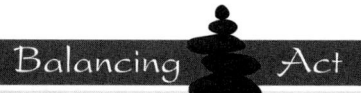

BREATHING EXERCISES

- Breathe in and hold your breath for a few seconds. Release and continue the process.

- Become aware of your breathing. As you exhale, try to breathe out even more slowly than you breathed in. Pause between exhalation and inhalation.

- Breathe in peace and joy. Each time you inhale, think about bringing peace rather than restlessness into your body. When you exhale, try to expel the restlessness within and around you. After doing this a few times, try to feel that you are breathing in joy and breathing out sorrow, suffering, and melancholy.

- Feel that you are breathing in cosmic energy to be used to purify your body. The energy is like a river flowing throughout your blood vessels. When you exhale, you are exhaling all of the impurities from your body, including thoughts and actions.

A good online resource for meditation is http://www. meditationworkshop.org/meditation_exercises. Most libraries have a good selection of meditation books. Find one that suits your needs and style best, and then make a commitment to practice meditation every day. Remember that one minute of meditation is better than no minutes of meditation.

Meditation is often prescribed as a way to lower blood pressure, improve exercise performance, breathe easier, relieve insomnia, and generally lessen the everyday stresses of life. It is a safe and simple way to balance a person's physical, emotional, and mental states. Anyone can benefit. Neuroscientists have found that those who meditate shift their brain activity to different areas of the cortex to become calmer. Jon Kabat-Zinn, PhD, recorded the brain waves of stressed employees of a high-tech firm in Madison, Wisconsin. The subjects were split randomly into two groups: 25 people were asked to learn meditation over 8 weeks, and the remaining 16 were left alone as a control group. All participants had their brain waves scanned three times during the study: at the beginning of the experiment, when meditation lessons were completed 8 weeks later, and 4 months after that. The researchers found that those who meditated showed a pronounced shift in activity to the left frontal lobe. They were calmer and happier than before (Davidson et al., 2003).

Using meditation for alleviating suffering and promoting healing is not new. Meditative techniques are the product of diverse cultures and peoples and are rooted in the traditions of the world's great religions. Meditation has become a valued part of complementary and alternative modalities in the West.

PRIMORDIAL SOUND MEDITATION

Primordial Sound Meditation (PSM) is a meditation technique in which practitioners repeat a mantra—a sound or vibration—to help achieve deeper awareness of self.

PSM is derived from the yoga tradition of India. Yoga means union—the union of environment, senses, body, mind, and soul. This union is described in an ancient text known as the Yoga Sutras, written by the sage Patanjali, in which he explains that yoga is the progressive settling down of the mind into the field of pure silence, which is usually overshadowed by the activity of the mind. When we access the silent spaces between thoughts, we enter the field of unbounded awareness.

The silence we experience is actually the gap between our thoughts. By enhancing our awareness of the gap, we recognize that our essential self is not the perpetual traffic of thoughts, but rather the silent witness to our thoughts, words, and actions. Regular practice of PSM promotes inner quietness in life, providing access to creativity and enabling us to make life-affirming choices.

Those who practice Hinduism believe past actions (karmas) create memories that generate desires (sanskaras) that lead to new actions (vasanas). The seeds of these memories and desires are present at the level of our soul, propelling each of us to make choices that define our lives. Meditation helps us recognize that we can make conscious choices that enable us to experience greater peace, love, success, and fulfillment. By reducing stress and fatigue, meditation helps us connect with our higher self—where energy, creativity, and inner awareness are our natural state of being.

QUANTUM LEAPS

What are you willing to settle for? Do you want a personal breakthrough or more of the same? You are working on simplifying and uncluttering. You have come to grips with yourself through meditation. Now you can leverage your performance to a new level. Prepare for a quantum leap. Timing is everything.

The Man Who Thinks He Can
—Walter D. Wintle

If you think you are beaten, you are;
If you think you dare not, you don't;
If you'd like to win, but think you can't,
It's almost a cinch you won't.
If you think you'll lose, you're lost,
For out in the word we find
Success begins with a fellow's will,
It's all in the state of mind.

If you think you're outcasted, you are;
You've got to think high to rise.
You've got to be sure of yourself before
You can ever win a prize.
Life's battles don't always go
To the stronger or faster man;
But sooner or later the man who wins
Is the man who thinks he can.

This poem is attributed to Walter D. Wintle, who lived in the late 19th and early 20th centuries. The first known publication date of the poem is 1905. It was published in *Poems That Live Forever*, compiled by Hazel Felleman, 1965.

If you keep on doing what you have done in the past, chances are you will achieve the same results. If you try harder at doing the same thing, you may make an incremental gain, but not a quantum leap. More of the same is a trap. To truly switch gears, you need to recognize that what you do is more important than how you do it.

Balancing Act

HUMANS BEING MORE

In a personal development class titled "Humans Being More," there is an exercise called "Getting to Japan." In this case, Japan is an arbitrary destination—it could just as easily be Hawaii, London, or Australia. Participants stand in a single line between two chairs and act out how they will get to Japan. This is a silent exercise; thus, the acting is intense. By imitating a plane, a hang-glider, a dance step, a train, or a swim stroke, participants convey the means of "transportation" to others in the room. The key is that the same method cannot be used more than once; participants must consistently be thinking outside of the box for new ways, new methods, to reach their destination. The end result—arriving in Japan—is the same for all players. How they got there—the method—does not matter, but the intention does matter. Think of it this way: When the intention is clear, the mechanism will appear. Intention plus mechanism equals results.

Our strengths often become our weaknesses because we rely on them too heavily, habitually doing what we do best instead of seeking the best things to do. For example, we may choose to travel to Japan by plane because that is the method we are most familiar with. Abraham Maslow once said, "If your only tool is a hammer, you tend to see every problem as a nail." Put down the hammer and find either a new tool or a different way to use that hammer. How we perceive problems is influenced by what tools we have for dealing with them. Today many people hammer away at issues, hoping to create major change with minimal chaos. That is like doing the same thing and expecting different results. Unfortunately, many of us are wired that way.

If we can begin to think outside of the box and beyond the hammer and nail mentality, we can find new ways to do things. We can create new ways to reach our goals—or get to Japan! Rather than continue the cycle of repetitiveness, we can become more aware of our intentions, alter our mechanisms, and change our results (www.nikken.com).

It's in your power. Make a quantum leap and achieve a personal breakthrough!

THE LAW OF ATTRACTION

The concept of the law of attraction is extremely simple: We attract whatever we choose to give our attention to—whether wanted or unwanted. It does not matter who you are, where you live, what your religious beliefs are, or in what year you were born. It is true for everyone equally. Once you "get it," there is no looking back. It will be part of you forever. Although promoted in *The Secret*, this law has been handed down through history. Great thinkers—Plato, Aristotle, Socrates, Michelangelo, Newton, Franklin, Jefferson, and many others—knew this tenet of life.

"With both trepidation and relief, J abandoned pragmatism in favor of magnetism."

—Tama Kieves

The simplest definition of this law is *like attracts like*. Other definitions include:

- You get what you think about, whether wanted or unwanted. You think that things will be negative, and they will. You think that things will be positive, and they will.
- You are a living magnet.
- You get what you put your energy and focus on, whether wanted or unwanted.
- Energy attracts like energy.

Experiment with it. If you normally think negatively, decide that you will spend one whole day thinking positively. Pay close attention and track the subtle and not-so-subtle differences. Consider as you go along that you have a choice as to how you react to everything that happens to you.

Keeping Your Balance
YOUR BALANCE SCORECARD

You can't walk the pathway to balance unless you understand where you currently stand. Complete the survey below to get an idea of where your strengths and weaknesses lie. Implement some of the ideas in this book, and then, a few months from now, retake the survey and see how you have improved.

MY BALANCE SCORECARD

1. How would you describe your current weight?

   ___Normal ___Overweight

2. How would you describe your current exercise level?

   ___Active ___Inactive

3. If you do not exercise, what is your main reason?

   ___Time ___Energy

4. How many hours of sleep did you get last night?

   ___Less than 6 ___More than 7

5. How many 8-ounce glasses of water do you drink a day?

   ___Less than 8 ___More than 8

6. Do you have problems with focus?

   ___Yes ___No

7. Describe your current energy level.

   ___High ___Low

8. How would you describe your motivation to eat healthy?

   ___Good ___Poor

9. How would you describe your morale?

   ___Good ___Poor

10. What factor plays the greatest part in your overall health?

    ___Self-motivation   ___Time

    ___Employer support   ___Money

11. Do you meditate?

    ___Yes ___No

12. Are you a "collector" of things/stuff/items that you do not necessarily need?

    ___Yes ___No

13. Do you powernap to relieve stress?

    ___Yes ___No

Date _____

*"Sometimes it seems your ever-increasing list
of things to do can leave you feeling totally
undone."*

—Susan Mitchell and Catherine Christie

3

STRESS

We hear about stress every day. It affects both our minds and our bodies. Job stress increases the risk of cardiovascular disease and the development of back and upper-extremity musculoskeletal disorders. The differences in rates of mental health problems, such as depression and burnout, for different occupations may be partly due to differences in job stress level. Clearly, we can reap significant benefits from reducing the stress in our lives at work and home.

But before we can create a formula for stress relief, we need to better understand the complex phenomena causing our hearts to be over-stimulated, our immune systems to be suppressed, our hormonal output to be unbalanced, and our reproductive systems to function abnormally.

WHAT IS THIS THING CALLED STRESS?

The physiology of stress can be described as a specific response by the body to a stimulus, such as pain or fear, that disturbs or interferes with the normal physiological equilibrium of an organism.

Stress is not unusual or abnormal. It's an everyday response by the body to an event. Your heart rate and respiration increase in anticipation of muscular activity. Stress is what your body experiences as it adjusts to ever-changing circumstances.

As a positive influence, stress can fill you with excitement and propel you into action or provide you with a feeling of happiness. Stress can be very motivating. It allows you to accomplish tasks and set goals and see them through to completion. This "good" stress is associated with the release of adrenaline, endorphins, serotonin, and dopamine, all of which act as natural antidepressants and pain relievers in the body.

> "Tension is who you think you should be.
> Relaxation is who you are."
> —Chinese Proverb

The body is amazing: It pumps adrenaline through our systems in response to stress, but if we do not use it up, that same adrenaline will manifest itself negatively in stress-induced tension, muscle pain, and more. Thus, a natural cycle within our bodies both relieves and contributes to stress.

STRESS AND CHOLESTEROL LEVELS

A negative reaction to stress can be seen in cholesterol levels. Stress may raise cholesterol levels, both immediately and over the long term. British researchers evaluating the stress reactions of 199 healthy adult men and women found that participants who reacted more strongly to emotional situations also demonstrated immediate and significant increases in cholesterol levels (Steptoe & Brydon, 2005). Three years later, these same study participants who initially responded more dramatically to stressful situations experienced a more significant elevation in cholesterol levels than other study participants. How significant? Those who had initial stress responses in the top third of the group were, 3 years later, more likely to have readings above the recommended levels for cholesterol than participants whose initial stress responses fell in the bottom third.

So, what is the stress-cholesterol connection? While researchers aren't certain, one theory is that stress might increase the body's inflammatory processes, which, in turn, increase lipid production.

WORKPLACE STRESS

Longer hours, greater workloads, staff reductions: These and other factors contribute to stress in the workplace. A healthy workplace helps combat stress.

"Men, for the sake of getting a living, forget to live."

—Margaret Fuller

"Workplace wellness" is a holistic concept that touches on many aspects of an organization and how it is managed. Successful workplace health and well-being programs are supported by senior management and form an integral part of the organization's strategy. Comprehensive workplace wellness plans typically comprise a range of programs and activities related to physical environment, health practices, and social environment.

A growing body of research indicates that workplace health and wellness initiatives have positive implications for both organizations and staff. Studies have found that implementation of wellness programs can result in better health for employees and lower health care costs for organizations.

A simple example of a wellness initiative is offering chair massage at no or reduced charge to employees. My former employer offered it on a monthly basis, and there was always a waiting list for this amazing, stress-reducing treatment.

REDUCING YOUR STRESS

Work isn't the only source of stress; our home lives can be just as hectic as our work lives. We need to reduce and manage stress at work and home. The body and mind need more short periods of rest than we allow. Just a few minutes of total relaxation will refresh you, so you can more effectively complete the task at hand. And yes, you can learn to fully relax for a few minutes a day in your home or even in your office setting.

"Don't underestimate the value of Doing Nothing, of just going along, listening to all the things you can't hear, and not bothering."

—Pooh's Little Instruction Book, inspired by A.A. Milne

One strategy we can use is the power nap. In a study of 23,681 participants who were free of coronary heart disease, stroke, or cancer at the time of enrollment, researchers found that a regular nap reduced coronary mortality. For example, those who napped on a regular basis (at least three times a week for an average of at least 30 minutes) had a 37% lower coronary mortality compared to those who did not rest. Working men had the highest benefit (Naska, Oikoniomou, Trichopoulou, Psaltopoulou, & Trichopoulos, 2007).

A power nap will put you into a refreshing phase of sleep, but not so deep that you wake up feeling even more tired than before. A power nap should last from a few minutes up to a maximum of 20 minutes and can be done anywhere that's safe and appropriate.

"Sometimes the most important thing in a whole day is the rest we take between two deep breaths."

—Etty Hillesum

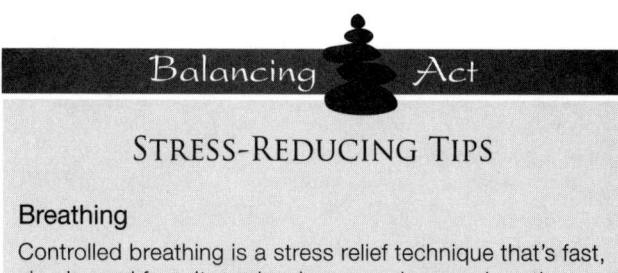

Balancing Act

STRESS-REDUCING TIPS

Breathing

Controlled breathing is a stress relief technique that's fast, simple, and free. It can be done anywhere and anytime, and it has numerous positive effects on your health, such as reducing high blood pressure.

Here's how basic controlled breathing works:

- Sit or stand in a relaxed position.
- Slowly inhale through your nose. Fill your lungs with fresh air and let your abdomen expand outward, rather than raising your shoulders.

- Exhale slowly through your mouth. Pay attention to the exhale. Drag it out for as long as possible.

- Repeat this exercise over 2 or 3 minutes and feel the tension release from your body.

Exercise

The human body needs to exercise to function properly. Exercise helps you think with more clarity, gives you more energy, and helps prevent diseases such as stroke and type 2 diabetes (Sarnataro, 2005).

It's a good idea to stretch before starting an exercise activity.

Stretching

My Cavalier King Charles Spaniel is a wonderful companion. He is 8 years old and very royal (or he thinks he is!). He just wants to be loved and to be near people. One of his morning rituals involves stretching. Not unlike a cat, he stretches his entire body—relieving stress in the process and preparing for a good morning walk. You can do the same thing! Stretch from the fingertips to the toes, including the face (yawning takes care of that). Be careful not to over-stretch, though, especially after long periods of inactivity. Stretching should not hurt. Affirmations are helpful. Write the word STRETCH on a sticky note and affix it to the computer monitor frame. Look at it often and take the hint to gently stretch the muscles and tendons in your fingers, wrists, neck, shoulders, back, and legs.

Simple Exercises

Walking is a very simple exercise and an excellent stress-relief technique. It doesn't require a lot of focus and can easily be incorporated into your workday, no matter how pressed for time you are. Take a brisk walk around the block, through your workplace, or up and down the stairs. Use up the adrenaline that's going through your bloodstream before it negatively impacts your health.

Sleep

We now know the benefits of a power nap. A 15-30 minute nap in the afternoon increases alertness, improves cognitive functioning, and reduces stress (Scott, 2008).

Adequate night-time sleep is also important. The body needs 8 hours per night, every night. The effects of lost sleep are cumulative and can result in impaired reaction time, vision, information processing, and short-term memory (Scott, 2008).

Eat Well

Eat well-balanced meals and take appropriate vitamins and minerals to make sure your body is adequately nourished and healthy. See Chapter 7, "Eat, Sleep, and Be Merry" for more on sleep and a balanced life.

Maintain a healthy body fat-to-muscle ratio. If necessary, concentrate on losing fat instead of just losing weight. Skinny does not equal healthy. The starlets who influence teenagers are not role models for health. When one loses weight quickly, that weight is easily regained, plus more. Starvation causes muscle loss and can contribute to weakness and serious illness.

Posture

Because adolescent girls hit their growth spurt earlier than boys, they sometimes slouch to avoid appearing taller. When I was a teenager, I remember parents reminding their daughters to sit upright, stand tall, and be proud of their height. The same adage continues to be true today. Remind yourself to maintain proper posture. If you sit most of the time, adjust the chair according to your body proportions. Keep your feet flat on the floor. Your rib cage should not rest on your hip joints.

Straighten your spine but don't hyperextend. Move your shoulders back, and take pressure off the spine in your neck by keeping your head aligned with the rest of the spine. I find that the use of a magnetized chair pad helps relieve pressure on the spine, and it improves my circulation at the same time.

Prioritize

Not everything needs to be taken care of right now. Recognize the difference between what is urgent and what is important, and manage your time wisely. Learn to say "no." Remind yourself that "no" is a complete sentence. Accept help when it's offered, or ask for help if you feel overwhelmed.

Keeping Your Balance

AN EXERCISE PLAN

How much time can you commit this week to exercise?
Next week? Use the grid to develop a regular schedule.
Try to build up to exercise at least 4 to 5 days per week.
Vary the type of exercise you do so you do not get bored
with your regimen.

	Monday	Tuesday	Wednesday	Thursday	Friday	Saturday	Sunday
Week 1							
Week 2							
Week 3							
Week 4							
Week 5							
Week 6							

Take a Power Nap

To jumpstart the power nap process, relax all the muscles of your body from the top of your head down to your toes. Imagine yourself in a warm and comfortable environment that has happy, relaxing memories for you, and gently will yourself into a relaxing sleep. Commit to yourself and you will drift into a gentle sleep.

You may think drifting into a relaxed state of being at your desk or elsewhere—as long as it's safe and appropriate— is impossible, but it will come easily with practice and concentrated effort.

You may question whether you will come out of this phase of sleep in a timely manner, but you will learn to set your own internal alarm clock that will wake you up at the right time. And, when you awaken, you will be refreshed and alive with vigor. Until you become proficient at power napping, feel free to set an alarm to remind you to wake up. However, select a gentle alarm bell so that you aren't jarred awake and lose the benefit of the restful feelings from the power nap. Better yet, partner with a friend to watch over each other to be sure you awaken on time.

The power nap relaxation exercises may be used throughout the day to fully relax your body. Simply relax all of your muscles from head to toe. Try it while sitting at your desk—loosen your neck and shoulders.

"In your thirst for knowledge, be sure not to drown in all the information."

—Anthony J. D'Angelo

4

PUTTING TECHNOLOGY IN ITS PLACE

Does technology help us, or is technology another form of information overload? Do you really need to know every detail, be part of every meeting, or read every piece of information you come across? Technology should support and enable your home and business processes, not dictate how your life is run. It's up to you to control how you use technology and not let the technology control you.

TECHNOLOGY CAN BE TOO MUCH OF A GOOD THING

Technology has simplified and complicated our lives. From electronic records to text messaging, our lives have changed and can sometimes seem to be controlled by bits and bytes. In an instant, we can send an e-mail message telling everyone on the "To" list the exact same thing at the exact same time. (Don't we all know someone who hit "send" on a "reply all" e-mail message and instantly regretted it?) Before, it was one postal letter at a time or one phone call at a time. We took the time to proofread and double check our work or words. We can also IM (instant message), text, Twitter, blog, write on our or someone else's Facebook wall, tag (their photos), and receive endless RSS (Rich Site Summary) feeds. In sum, we have far more contact with far more people and information on a daily basis than ever before in human history. This can create unnecessary stress in our lives when we try to keep up with everything.

"Technology ... is a queer thing. It brings you great gifts with one hand, and it stabs you in the back with the other."

–C.P. Snow, New York Times, 15 March 1971

Balancing Act

"OUI, ALLÔ": A HOME CARE NURSE AND TECHNOLOGY

In Quebec, a French province in Canada, the alarm went off when it seemed to be way too early. It was still dark outside and the wind was howling. Jolted from her dream, Nicole jumped up to the alarm blazing Beethoven's 5th Symphony. "Michel," she thought. Her son understood all of the new technology. She couldn't even set her own alarm clock.

She hurried to get ready for what was to be a busy schedule. She had mapped out her route the night before to get a head start. Suddenly, the phone rang.

"Oui, Allô."

It was the office.

Knowing that Nicole had an early start, Gillian, who organizes life in home care from the office, said, "I'm glad I caught you. We've just had a call from someone who sounds quite upset. Her mother, Mrs. Quinn, is 89 years old and lives alone. Because she lives out of town, the daughter calls her often. Mrs. Quinn hasn't sounded great these last few days and the daughter is worried. Can you give her a call? She wonders if you can visit her mom and call her with some feedback."

Taking down the details, Nicole added her to the list. She was afraid to try entering the information into her new Blackberry—just another new gadget to learn to use. It was on another list of things to do, but not today!

First stop was Mrs. Jansen. She is diabetic and needed bloodwork drawn before the meal. Mrs. Jansen lives alone and loves the nurses' visits.

"Stay for tea," she said.

Nicole thought about everything she had to do and hesitated for just a moment before agreeing.

"A quick tea and hold the donut," Mrs. Jansen added. Nicole smiled, noticing the twinkle in her eye, and pulled up a chair.

On the road again, sitting in her car, Nicole called the distraught daughter from out of town.

"My mother sounds terrible this morning, and she can't explain how she is doing. I have been noticing changes, and she seems to forget what we have been talking about. I am really worried about her, and she won't go to the doctor."

Nicole decided that she should visit this woman's mom and asked the daughter to tell her mother that someone was coming to see her. Nicole added Mrs. Quinn to her list. If only she could enter the information into her Blackberry, it would save her time later. Another list, another day, all in good time she thought.

As Nicole greeted her next patient, Mrs. Germaine, she remembered why she stayed in nursing.

"Hi, Mrs. Germaine. I am here to help get you more comfortable. You've had a tough night."

There were obvious signs of pain. Nicole quickly checked the medication records to see what she had been given. After giving Mrs. Germaine an additional morphine dose, she quietly sat, holding her hand until the grimace softened and her breathing eased.

Nicole continued to try to make Mrs. Germaine more comfortable by massaging her legs and back. "Have you ever been to a spa?" she asked. She knew the probable answer, because Mrs. Germaine was a nurse who was well known in the community for spending every available hour helping others. "No, I never have," she said. "Then let's imagine that this is your day at the spa." A tear fell down Mrs. Germaine's cheek, and she smiled. "It feels wonderful," she said, as she dozed off to sleep.

Just as Nicole was getting in her car after the visit with Mrs. Germaine, the phone rang.

"Oui, Allô." It was Gillian from the office again. "Mr. Desmarais has called four times this morning. He sounds more and more anxious, and he says that he is sweating." There was no real panic in Gillian's voice. Mr. Desmarais had done this before, and it usually was because he got nervous as the time approached for his caregiver to arrive. He wanted to make sure she was coming and that the same caregiver that he likes had been assigned. "No changes!" he would say. "If you have to send someone different, don't send anyone." Typically, Gillian reassured him by telling him that the time would be as scheduled and that Carol, his favourite nurse, would be there. Today, though, Gillian could not calm him and called Nicole for back-up.

Nicole had his number in one of her tech gadgets but did not trust that she could find it quickly. In the name of expediency, she took his number from Gillian and agreed to call him. Mr. Desmarais' anxiety disorder made it difficult for him to cope at times. Nicole hoped a phone call would do. Mr. Desmarais knew her well after several visits and was happy to hear her voice. He repeated what he had said to Gillian. Nicole reminded him about the breathing exercises they had practiced. She did some exercises on the phone with him. She was convinced that he had worked himself up and now seemed to be calming down with her talking and breathing with him. "Carol will be there in 1 hour. Will you be OK?" "I think so," he said with some hesitation.

Mrs. Quinn, the lady with the daughter from out of town, was next, because she lived close to where Nicole was at that time. She was also not sure what she would find and wanted to get back to the daughter as soon as possible. She rang the doorbell.

"Her daughter was supposed to tell her I was coming," Nicole thought, but so far, no answer. Nicole was aware of the fact that so often parents do not want their children telling them what to do and that they are just fine, "thank you very much." She respected that and tried not to be judgmental and to understand their position.

It was freezing out! Oh, please open the door. She looked up and saw an elderly woman peering through the window. The woman shook her head, mouthing the words, "Not today, thank you."

Back to the car and on the phone with Mrs. Quinn's daughter.

"It is hard to tell from out here, but she looks OK at this moment. She is standing and talking and politely informing me that my presence is not welcome today. We can call her again later. Maybe she will accept a visit tomorrow. If you are still concerned, you can call 911. We have seen this so often. People who are independent all of their lives still want to do things their way."

She hung up and heard the beep telling her she had a message to call the office.

"Oui, Allô. C'est Nicole."

"Mark called to confirm your visit. He said he knows he set the time for 2 p.m., but he wonders if you can come a bit earlier." Yes, of course she would.

The next visit was a challenge. The house was in a state of disarray, and although Nicole was accustomed to similar situations, it never ceased to amaze her that people live in the most challenging conditions. The patient valued her independence and did not want others, including her son, to interfere. Frail and obviously suffering, the patient finally agreed to go to the hospital to ease her discomfort. Nicole called for an ambulance. The patient passed away in the hospital, in no pain, and with her son at her bedside.

Again, her phone rang. "Oui, Allô." It was her son reminding her that she promised to pick him up because his car was in the garage. "Mom, I texted you." Frustrated, she told him she could read it but couldn't reply. Just as she thought she could learn the two-thumb typing tango after her first practice with him, strange things happened. She'd punched three clicks for the third letter and the word "big" would appear or "Hi." That's not what she wanted. It was as if the phone was trying to guess what she wanted to say. She gave up. "I need another lesson. I will be there at 6 p.m. If you want me to get you to hockey practice tomorrow morning, set my alarm for 6 a.m. I can't figure it out and have no time to learn it tonight."

The phone rang again. "Oui, Allô." As she listened, she became confused. It sounded like one of her clients on her list today but the client, Susan, usually called through the office. Her very distinctive voice and usual "I'm not happy" sound was loud and clear, though.

And then there was a snicker. Nicole realized it was Gillian, who was so accustomed to the frequent calls from Susan that she could sound just like her. Gillian laughed as she realized she had done her job well. Lightening Nicole's day, she just wanted to ask if Nicole could visit Susan earlier, as Susan had called the office complaining about one of her caregivers and wanted help getting organized for the adaptive van scheduled to take her to the Day Center. She was on Nicole's list anyway, so off she went.

Nicole's greeting from Susan as she walked through the door was: "Why did it take you so long to get here? What kind of caregivers do you have? You know I can't do things for myself and they do it all wrong!"

Nicole had heard this many times in the year that they had been caring for Susan. How sad that she was all alone, in bed, and mobile only because of her electric wheelchair and some adaptive devices. These gave her freedom—freedom to be in charge of one small part of her life. Freedom to get around if properly set up with ankle supports and controls in hand. Freedom to live a little. Nicole knew that she'd have to talk to the staff again, to try to help them understand Susan's frustration, anger, and fear. Susan also had to understand how the caregivers feel, often being "kicked out" even when they really try to do things Susan's way.

She was up for it, but first Susan needed help to get organized for her outing. Nicole was amazed at how well Susan was able to cope once she was organized and happier. She had the door to her apartment fitted with a rope to close it on her way out, told the cats to go to their room and they listened. She managed the electric controls on her wheelchair, almost doing wheelies in the hall, and off she went. Nicole thought about how much we could learn from Susan every day.

"I'll try to be nice tomorrow when Marlene comes," she shouted as the elevator doors closed.

Darkness and cold wind accompanied her home. By 10 p.m., after picking up Michel, having dinner, and doing some prepping for the next evening, she started to feel the effects of her long day. She was wiped out. Sleep came easily to Nicole. She was lucky that way. Life got sorted out and seemed to make sense most of the time, except when she woke from a deep sleep, startled.

"Did I forget to call the doctor for Mrs. Jane's appointment?"

And then she remembered that Gillian took care of it and she drifted back to sleep. That dream again … the list. Where is it? She has lost it.

"No," she laughed in her dream, "I know where it is and it just keeps getting longer."

It didn't worry her anymore. She hid it away for a little longer. It was like her private little joke. At 6 a.m. the alarm went off—this time to "Oh Canada." Oh, that clown Michel. And so the day began. Nicole's phone rang as she was heading out the door with her son for his hockey practice. "Oui, Allô."

THE PRACTICAL SIDE OF TECHNOLOGY

While technology can seem to complicate our lives with a glut of information and electronic demands, it has also simplified our lives by allowing us to be organized, on time, and on task. Can you manage technology without having it manage you? Of course! But first people need to understand how to manage themselves. A Blackberry or other personal digital assistant (PDA) will be of no benefit if you consistently check e-mail and ignore the work that needs to be done. More gadgets often call for more discipline. Think of technology as if the electronic files were paper files, continuously stacking up on your desk waiting to be processed.

Also take advantage of all the practical features of most e-mail software packages. Most offer some form of electronic calendar, task lists, sticky notes, flags for follow-up and organizing, e-mail reminders, and rules for automatically sorting and filing e-mails. For example, if you work with specific team members on a project, and the only e-mails you get from those team members relate to that project, you can tell your software to automatically send those messages to a folder that you will then manage during time set aside for that project. If your business or community education services offer courses on managing e-mail software, take advantage of them to learn the best approaches to manage your technology tools.

Your goal should be to manage content without chaos. Don't allow the technology to rule your life. Instead, allow the technology to contribute to work/life balance by making your time yours alone.

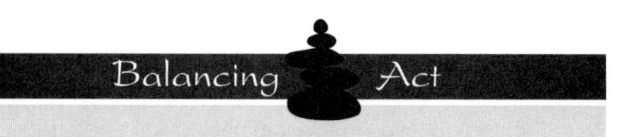

Balancing Act

TAME YOUR E-MAIL

Many people check their e-mail even when they do not have time to handle everything in their inbox. Instead of this approach, only check e-mails during times you have set aside for handling them, never when you're rushing off or have just a few minutes before a meeting. When you do check your e-mail, read and handle the messages then. When looking at e-mail, one of four decisions can be made:

1. Review the message once and act on it; either delete it, file it, or forward it.

2. If a quick response is all that is needed, do it now and move on.

3. If needed, delegate the task to someone else.

4. If the e-mail is project- or task-based, schedule a reminder via your e-mail software to trigger an alert when due.

Keeping Your Balance

Are you master of technology such as e-mail and cell phones, or is technology the master of you? Try this self-assessment to see where you fall.

Answer each question yes or no.

1. I organize myself before placing a telephone call.

2. I schedule telephone conversations to avoid playing phone tag.

3. If I have a complicated question, I call the person instead of sending an e-mail.

4. If I am exchanging multiple e-mails on a single issue, I call instead of continuing to e-mail.

5. I set time to respond to my e-mail instead of interrupting my work for each one.

6. I keep my contacts list up to date with e-mail, phone, and fax, so I can easily contact those I need to reach.

7. I use an electronic calendar to keep track of my appointments.

8. I update my voicemail and e-mail, so people can reach me before problems get out of hand.

9. I turn off my cell phone (or put it on vibrate if I'm expecting an important call) when at a restaurant.

10. I take the appropriate time to learn new technology systems or devices *before* trying to implement them.

The more "yeses," the more you are in control of technology.

Excerpted from Pagana, K.P., 2008.

"Care enough for a result, and you will almost certainly attain it."

—William James

5

FOCUS

Our chaotic lives can easily distract us from our focus. How many times in a day do you find yourself in a room, knowing you were there for a reason, but unable to remember the reason you went there? Or, at the end of the day with a heavy sigh, you look over your to-do list from that morning and realize you barely made a dent in your list? We joke and attribute it to old age—even the young do this—but more likely it is a difficulty in maintaining focus.

Focus is the thing that keeps us on track. It's what we do when we have a goal to achieve. We keep *focused* on doing what we need to do to accomplish the tasks that cumulatively make up the goal. Focus is also an ability to remain undistracted. It is what we use to intently pursue a goal like running the Boston Marathon, studying for exams, writing a paper, or creating artwork. It is this kind of focus that is the source of the "Ah-Ha" moment we hope for when seeking solutions and setting goals. Getting to it, to that Ah-Ha moment of achievement or recognition, includes the knowledge of how to define *your* path and work *your* plan.

"Chance favors only the prepared mind."

—Louis Pasteur

Ah-Ha! How often do you say this? Is it the time when you have thought of something new or suddenly been blessed with a moment of inspiration? We are all familiar with these moments, but we cannot predict when they will come. Sometimes it takes days and hours of focus, and sometimes just a few minutes. Sometimes it's much longer and evolves through trial and error and contributions from external sources.

Focus is facilitated through good health. Health is about mind and body. If your consciousness is disturbed, then your body will be too. If you are uptight, your body will be tense and it will be difficult to focus. So how do you keep your focus so that you experience more of those Ah-Ha moments? Consider the following strategies:

- Be centered
- Tap into your creative side
- Keep the "main thing" the main thing
- Set goals and write them down
- Find your passion

Balancing Act

AN AH-HA MOMENT: ARCHIMEDES IN THE BATH

The story of Archimedes in the bath illustrates just such an Ah-Ha moment. The king, Hiero, having requested a special crown be made, delivered a certain weight in gold to the crown maker. Upon receiving his crown, some suspicion was raised as to whether or not the crown maker had replaced some of the gold with an equal weight of another metal and kept the extra gold for himself—stealing the king's gold. The king asked Archimedes to prove the content of the crown. Archimedes, entering into his bath, was suddenly struck with the idea that his body weight displaced the water in the tub. Taking this as the beginning of his discovery, it is said that he made two masses of the same weight as the crown, one of gold and the other of silver. After making them, he filled a large vessel with water to the very brim, and dropped the mass of silver into it. As much water ran out as was equal in bulk to that of the silver sunk in the vessel. Then, taking out the mass, he poured back the lost quantity of water, using a pint measure, until it was level with the brim as it had been before. Thus he found the weight of silver corresponding to a definite quantity of water. After this experiment, he likewise dropped the mass of gold into the full vessel and, on taking it out and measuring as before, found that not so much water was lost, but a smaller quantity: Specifically, a mass of gold lacks in bulk compared to a mass of silver of the same weight. Finally, filling the vessel again and dropping the crown itself into the same quantity of water, he found that more water ran over for the crown than for the mass of gold of the same weight. Hence, reasoning from the fact that more water was lost in the case of the crown than in that of the mass, he detected the mixing of silver with the gold, and made the theft of the contractor perfectly clear.

BE CENTERED

Being centered means not letting yourself be overshadowed by what's going on around you. If you're not centered, you will be like a yo-yo at the mercy of circumstance; you will be out of focus.

> When you start on that action, and a "distraction" pops up, there's a little conversation that goes on in your head. And in that conversation you make a choice: You either settle for giving

up working on the task at hand, or you stand
up for yourself and say, "I'm not willing to
give up working on this worthy goal for this.
I'm not willing to settle for less."

This is a big deal. It's bigger than willpower.
It's bigger than raw motivation. It's simply the
willingness to cling to how important your goal
is and how much less important a distraction
is. Because when you can put the two actions
in perspective relative to each other, you can
make focus a no-brainer activity. (Navarro,
2006, ¶8-9)

"Knowledge is power."

—Sir Francis Bacon

During those Ah-Ha moments, you are charged up and your
mind is working optimally. During those moments, you can be
all that you wish to be—creative, centered, focused. One of
the most important ladders leading to the top is knowledge.
The more we know, the more prepared our mind is, and the
higher we can move. You need to make sure that your mind is
prepared and that you are focused. When we are centered, we
are more receptive to new ideas and knowledge.

Balancing Act

THE SPELLING BEE

Our son, at age 12, was preparing for the National Spelling Bee. He was always a good speller, but he focused on the fact that in order to win the prize, a computer, he would need to outspell all other contestants. Working with his coach, an English teacher, he accumulated all of the books used in previous years and a list of "difficult" words. He strategized on how many words he would have to study per night, over a 1-year period, in order to win the prize. I worked with him on a nightly basis, and our goal was to cover 200 words per night. Blessed with a photographic memory, he gave me many Ah-Ha moments. For example, I would say "antimacassar" and he said, "Is that page 3, the third column, fourth word?" Of course, he was correct—he was focused. But, not only could he remember the words as they appeared on the written page, he was able to tell me the origin and meaning, and spell each word accurately.

The qualifying rounds for Nationals were conducted at Trinity University, where he was seated behind a young boy from a small town in Texas. The boy said, "When I am finished here, my dad is going to take me fishing." Our son replied, "When I am finished here, I am going to go home and play with my new computer." Both boys were committed to a goal; both were focused, but our son was also focused on the prize. He went on to win the San Antonio Spelling Bee—and the computer.

When we arrived in Washington, DC, we were staggered by the number of winners from cities and states across the country, all of whom were good spellers. While all of the participants were focused on the Spelling Bee itself, many switched gears and focused on the excitement of their first airplane flight and the chance to see history come alive through the monuments and treasures of the nation's capitol. Many of these contestants, after they dropped out in the first and second rounds, went on sightseeing trips and took advantage of the opportunity for continuous learning through the sights and sounds of Washington, DC. Our son maintained his focus with a strong sense of balance, designating certain hours of the day for review of the words and other time slots for sightseeing. This, for me, was an Ah-Ha moment: A lesson from a 12-year-old boy on how to maintain balance in one's life.

TAP INTO YOUR CREATIVE SOUL

Imagination is seeing things not as they are, but as they could be. I have had the privilege of living in many cities and states, and for a short time, abroad. The concept of house hunting is not new to me. In the days before online searches of potential properties in the right school districts with the right soccer teams, I visited thousands of homes over the years. Fortunately, I was able to imagine what the homes would look like with my own special touches of paint, wall covering, new carpeting, and our own things. When we settled on a property, I used a four-step process, tapping into my creative soul—quite deeply at times—to bring these houses to life and make a house a home. The four steps are:

1. Preparation
2. Incubation
3. Illumination
4. Implementation

Those four steps may easily be transferred into many of our daily activities. When we approach a new project, we need to *prepare* by gathering information and resources. We then *incubate* the idea, letting our subconscious mind play with the information. Next, we experience the Ah-Ha moment, *illuminating* the idea and bringing it to life. And finally, we *implement*, either by doing or not doing a certain action or strategy. John Maxwell once said, "Lots of folks have great ideas in the shower, but they seem to lose them when they dry off." Is that you? It may be easier if you think about all the times in your career when you went through these steps to help a patient. Take the example of the nurse who wanted to help a lonely male resident at a long-term care facility. She prepared by gathering information about the man, his family (all living out of state), his past hobbies (writing, but he could no longer use a keyboard or pen), and past experiences (teaching). She let her information incubate until she had an Ah-Ha moment: The man narrated stories about his family into a tape recorder and sent them to his family, who copied the tapes and sent them back. He also started teaching other residents how to write their own memoirs.

"Over the years I have developed a picture of what a human being living humanely is like. She is a person who understands, values, and develops her body, finding it beautiful and useful; a person who is real and is willing to take risks, to be creative, to manifest competence, to change when the situation calls for it, and to find ways to accommodate to what is new and different, keeping that part of the old that is still useful and discarding what is not."

–Virginia Satir

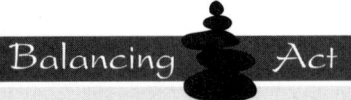

FIND YOUR MOTIVATION

All kinds of studies have been made regarding motivation. What is it that motivates people to do the things they do, live the way they live, achieve the goals they achieve? The root of the word motivation is *move*, and movement is change. Ask yourself: Are you moving forward or standing still? Do you love your work? Your career? Do you have good personal relationships? Is your attitude in check? Are you in balance?

Our comfort zones padlock the doors to growth, discovery, and adventure. Unlock those doors and focus on the prize. We don't remember days as much as we remember moments. Make the Ah-Ha moments count!

KEEP THE "MAIN THING" THE MAIN THING

What does that mean to you? The Ah-Ha moment is something you can't plan; it just comes. And, it is a joy to be there when that moment occurs for someone you know. Within nursing, we have many Ah-Ha moments, such as when students discover that the first bed bath is not that difficult, and as new graduates, when we discover the passion of our role within the profession. As a nurse educator, we see the smile on the face of a student and realize that he or she has connected the dots and that the complex process that we just explained is quite simple after all. Within nursing administration it may be when we realize that we have met our expectations for the organization and fulfilled our professional and personal goals.

"If you chase two rabbits, both will escape."
—Chinese Proverb

SET GOALS

At the start of every year, people all across the world set goals or resolutions for the New Year. Many of these resolutions are promises that all-too-often get broken—to lose 10 pounds, to increase exercise, to give up one bad habit or another, and to live a better life. Many of these resolutions are actual goals with commitments and action plans for success, many of which are executed successfully.

Yet, there are those of us who set goals, state affirmations, get motivated, and do not succeed. Are you one of them? In reality, a very small percentage of people actually set purposeful goals and follow them through.

It has often been said that the line that separates winning from losing is as fine as a razor's edge. One may *see* an opportunity and the other may *seize* an opportunity.

FIND YOUR PASSION

We want to feel passionate about the work that we do and define our contribution to mankind, our purpose for being. We want to know that we are contributing to the greater good and that our life has meaning, and that we contribute to the lives of those around us. We want to find our calling! But, do we know what that calling really is?

"Don't ask yourself what the world needs;
ask yourself what makes you come alive.
And then go and do that. Because what
the world needs is people who have come
alive."

—Harold Whitman

It would be so much easier if, during high school, we were
sent a directive for our life's work. It would be so much easier
if we went to university with a known major and maintained
that major through graduation. It would be so much easier if
our class schedule remained a constant, if our first selection
of an employer was the right one for us, and if our selection
of a life's partner was also the right one from the start. That
would certainly decrease the number of divorces. But, life is
not like that. And, we are not handed a directive that will last
throughout our lives. Instead, life is a process, and by going
through the process, we focus on an evolution of ourselves
through time.

A career in nursing is likewise a process, taking the nurse
from classroom to clinical area, from research to management,
and many other areas in between. Regardless of the clinical
setting in which care is given, the process is an evolution in
studying, caring, creating the evidence base, partnering with
patients and others to enhance outcomes, and celebrating our
successes. We might begin a career on a medical-surgical unit
and transition to the emergency department, intensive care,
pediatrics, operating room, or home care. And even within
the clinical setting, we might choose to specialize in oncology,
neurology, infusion therapy, maternal-child health, or ortho-
pedics.

"Passion is universal humanity. Without it religion, history, romance, and art would be useless."

—Honoré de Balzac

A BLUEPRINT FOR SUCCESS: FOCUS

Human beings come into this world to do particular work. Those of us in the health professions are here to do special work. Teachers provide a special gift to participate in molding young minds. The work is our purpose, and each is specific to the person. Focus is a blueprint for success, and by being focused on the goal, we position ourselves for success.

The search is an integral part of the process. Finding out who you are is one of the key steps in finding out what you are here to do. And, it may just be the most important step in keeping you focused. Who are you as a nursing professional? Where is your blueprint for success?

Keeping Your Balance

REFLECTION

- What was your last Ah-Ha moment? Think about the children you know. How often do they have Ah-Ha moments?

- Think about what helps you relax and tap into your creative side. Perhaps it's walking in the park, listening to hip hop, relaxing with a hot cup of tea, or writing in a journal. Once you identify what helps boost your creativity, you can plan more time for it.

- Think about a work-related goal you want to achieve and state your goal S.M.A.R.T.— specific, measureable, attainable, realistic, timely. Share the goal with a trusted colleague or friend who can help you develop steps to achieve the goal.

PART II
FINDING AND KEEPING BALANCE

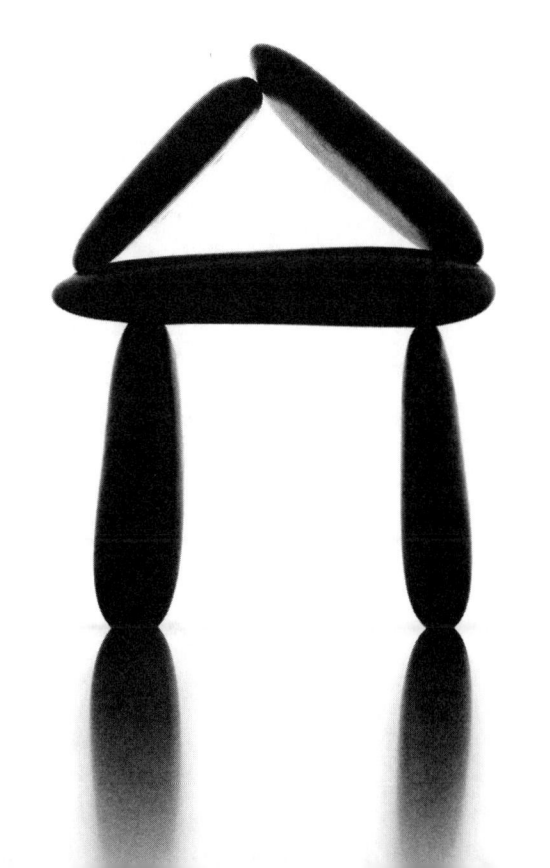

"Life is like riding a bike. It is impossible to maintain your balance while standing still."

—Linda Brakeall

6

WORKPLACE BALANCE

Good employers recognize the value of good employees, and they are often willing to find or create ways to help employees deal with family situations by making short-term or permanent changes in work schedules. Options include flextime, job-sharing, telecommuting, and part-time employment. If you know your skills, abilities, and performance record are strong and valued, you have a solid footing for negotiating flexible work arrangements.

What is negotiation? Practically, it's making the other person an offer or proposal that he or she may find more attractive than the next best alternative. Some consider negotiation to be the art of making deals. It is certainly that, but it also involves educating the other party about merits of your offer or proposal—or talents, skills, and actual and potential contributions. Negotiation is a key component of creating workplace balance and thus avoiding burnout. And, negotiation requires advance planning on your part. The process is simple, but each step is critical to the outcome.

1. Be prepared. Follow the tips and understand the rationale—know what you want and understand what the other party wants.

2. Open with your case; this demonstrates confidence. Then, listen actively.

3. Support your case with facts.

4. Explore areas of agreement and disagreement, and seek understanding and possibilities.

5. Indicate your readiness to work together.

6. Know your options.

7. Advance to closure by confirming the details.

8. Make it happen!

TIP	RATIONALE
Know what you are willing to accept, and have viable options.	You will be empowered in support of your interests. Your listener will recognize your confidence level.
Do not disclose what you are willing to accept (walk-away alternatives).	Disclosure will compromise your negotiating power.
Determine what the other party is willing to accept.	It is better to know the alternatives up-front than to second-guess.
Be an active listener, like a student.	Assume there are things about the situation that you don't understand. Let the other party know that you have heard and understood what has been said.

BURNOUT

If you are a busy person with a demanding job and family and friends who seek your time and attention, you are blessed, but *only* if you can handle it. Working from home can be beneficial, because you can maintain some control over your schedule.

"People who cannot find time for recreation are obliged sooner or later to find time for illness."

—John Wanamaker

However, some busy people feel guilty regardless of what they are doing. They may feel guilty spending time with friends and family, because they are not getting work done. Likewise, when working intensely, they feel guilty because they're not paying attention to others or taking good care of themselves. That feeling can lead to burnout—when the stress lasts so long that your ability to function is impaired. Burnout symptoms include, but are not limited to:

Powerlessness	Feeling trapped
Hopelessness	Failure
Emotional exhaustion	Despair
Detachment	Cynicism
Isolation	Apathy
Irritability	

We hear a lot about burnout within the health care sector. Nurses work 12-plus hour shifts and endure long stretches without time off. The demand on time and talent is extreme. When staffing is an issue, nurses work longer hours. When the economy is at an all-time low, nurses work additional hours or multiple jobs to make ends meet.

Burnout can be prevented by following the advice of experts and those who have personally experienced burnout. The main point they make is that we benefit greatly by maintaining clear boundaries between our work lives and our personal lives.

ESTABLISH CLEAR BOUNDARIES

When your work life and personal life blend together under the guise of "multi-tasking," both suffer. When you are at work, focus on the job to be done. When you are finished with work, don't bring it home with you. Make time for your personal life. If your work materials are dispersed throughout nearly every room of your house, you have no place for a real retreat. You're not spending high-quality time with friends or family members if you're talking on your cell phone or checking your e-mail when you're with them. Take time to focus exclusively on your friends and family members when you're with them; then you won't feel guilty when you have to concentrate on work. Create high-quality work and personal experiences for yourself by keeping them separate.

"I arise in the morning torn between the desire to improve the world and a desire to enjoy the world. This makes it hard to plan the day."

—E.B. White

CREATE A DESIGNATED WORK AREA AT HOME

When you are in your home "office," that's the time to pay bills, answer letters, and reply to electronic mail. When you are finished, walk away from the office and computer. Instead of checking e-mail frequently, set aside specific time frames during the day. Then reward yourself with personal time.

BECOME AN EFFICIENCY EXPERT

If you negotiate a telecommuting arrangement, keep in mind that many professionals find it difficult to adjust to working from home. The freedom of working in casual clothing, of not reporting for work at a specific time, and of not being directly supervised by others creates an environment that may become lax. You must be responsible for your own efficiency, effectiveness, and efforts. Is your work environment efficient and ergonomically correct? Does it lend itself to a high level of productivity in a short time span? Are you a morning person—someone who works best in the early hours of the day? Set a schedule to plan your work at home, and then work according to your plan.

SCHEDULE TIME FOR MEALS, RELAXATION, AND EXERCISE

You schedule appointments with other people in your personal planner, so why not schedule time with yourself? Make appointments for regular exercise, a hearty walk, or meditation.

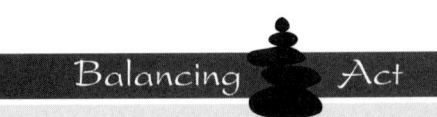

IF YOU MISS AN APPOINTMENT WITH YOURSELF ...

If you find that you don't have the discipline to keep the appointment with yourself, include a friend or family member in the healthy activity and make an appointment with them. It will be harder to postpone, and you'll have quality time with that person as a bonus.

KNOW WHAT IS IMPORTANT

In his book *The 7 Habits of Highly Effective People*, Stephen Covey showed that for many of us, the day is filled with tasks that attract our attention and seem urgent, but they may never need to be done. Weed those out and make time for the important tasks. The important duties that are also urgent require our immediate attention.

RECOGNIZE THE NEED FOR HELP AND GIVE IT BACK

If you are feeling burned out, you are not alone. In a Harris Interactive poll, 42% of those surveyed said they were currently struggling with job burnout (Harris Poll, 2005). In a CareerBuilder.com poll (2006), 77% reported sometimes feeling burned out. There are people who can help you. Share your feelings with friends and family, and let them pick up the ball when you need help. In turn, make it a practice to be of service to others and "pay it forward."

Also, consider helping others. Many people say that when they feel stressed, going out of their way to help someone else makes them feel better. Pay it forward, and change the world one good deed at a time.

KNOW YOUR LIMITATIONS

Are you an assertive type who finds it easy to say "no"? Or, are you a selfless type who takes on more than you can handle? Negotiate for workplace balance by knowing yourself and your limitations, and remember that "no" can be a complete sentence. This means that it's perfectly acceptable to say "no" without any further explanation. Nurses are notorious for putting the needs of others before their own. Perhaps part of the gratification nurses get from their job is being of service to others. To effectively care for others, you must center yourself. There are several centering techniques. Many involve being quiet and still with yourself—either sitting, walking, or absorbed in a hobby. You can find one that works for you. Practice your technique even when you feel great. It will help prevent stress and burnout.

Balancing Act

CENTERING YOURSELF

Leonard Orr originated a technique called conscious breathing that you can use to help center yourself. You can access a video of Orr's version (20 Connected Breaths) from http://www.rebirthingbreathwork.com/videoclips.

Tend to Your Own Interests

Winston Churchill said that a laborer benefits from physical rest and a sedentary person benefits from exercise. Those of us who deal with people can benefit by switching to an activity that absorbs the mind and makes it difficult to think about our problems for a while.

Try Something New

You may know that what you are doing now is not working well. Perhaps the balance between your work and personal life is off. Working harder at the same activities does not create balance. Consider changing your schedule or altering your routine to try to reset the balance. Exercise in the morning instead of after work. Find a combination that works best for you and that re-energizes your life.

In their book *Just Enough*, Laura Nash and Howard Stevenson showed through in-depth interviews, case studies, and surveys of top executives that successful people who found the greatest satisfaction in their lives paid attention to happiness, achievement, significance, and legacy throughout their entire lives. Nash and Stevenson recommend that we continually seek contentment and accomplishment, and that we focus on making a positive impact on people we care about and ways to help others find future success. We can do these things, and prevent burnout at the same time, by being mindful of how we're living moment to moment.

An important element of preventing burnout is the actual work environment. Whether we work independently or as members of a team and regardless of our clinical setting, people can and do make the difference!

HAVE THE RIGHT PEOPLE IN THE RIGHT SEATS ON THE BUS

Having a lot of help is not enough if it isn't the right help for the right job. Make a concerted effort to surround yourself with good people, and give them the latitude they need to do a good job. As an example, within the nursing community, having the right people in a busy emergency department (ED) will ensure appropriate triage, timely service, and quality outcomes. Because there is no such thing as the "average" day in the ED, members of the health care team can collectively:

- Define stretch targets for length of stay.
- Implement a monitoring system for status of patients in emergency departments to be reviewed at pre-defined intervals.
- Coordinate resources.
- See the right person at the right time.
- Fast-track patients as needed.
- Track communications with patients:

    Waiting to be seen,

    Waiting for admission,

    Waiting for discharge.

"In order that people may be happy in their work, these three things are needed: They must be fit for it. They must not do too much of it. And they must have a sense of success in it."

—John Ruskin

Another good example may be seen in an Institute for Healthcare Improvement initiative developed by a Florida Hospital, Orlando, Florida, team whose goal was to decrease door-to-door time in the emergency department.

The team, with the right key players in place, implemented the following strategic actions:

- **Predictive model:** They looked at the previous 4 weeks of volume, key metrics, and admissions and determined daily demand. Staffing is now consistent with demand.

- **Reduced lab turnaround:** They decreased time in getting specimens to the lab, thus facilitating receipt of results.

- **Looked for and decreased wasted or non-value-added steps:** They observed and videotaped processes and redesigned work areas to ensure closer proximity to patients.

- **Incorporated lean tools into daily process:** Two of the tools are single patient flow and simplifying tasks.

- **Developed a monthly process council:** Representation includes nursing and senior leadership. Following process review and outcomes, action plans are developed to help the team meet its goals.

Examples like these are easily applied to one's own clinical setting; they contribute to positive outcomes, staff satisfaction, and balance.

Working together, nurses can achieve successes unattainable by individuals. The knowledge that there are others around you who are pulling with you to attain a shared goal enhances the rewards of a professional nursing career.

FAMILY-FRIENDLY WORK ENVIRONMENTS

Family-friendly working and work/life balance refer to working arrangements that help us achieve a better balance between work and family life. These may include maternity and paternity leave, on-site child care, flextime, job sharing, working from home, and other creative solutions.

"When people go to work, they shouldn't have to leave their hearts at home."

—Betty Bender

RE-ENTERING THE WORKFORCE

If you are re-entering the workforce after taking time off, your preference may be to work part time or have a flexible schedule. If your priorities in life require that you have a flexible work schedule or work part time, you should inform a potential employer of those expectations during the interview process. Otherwise, you may be dissatisfied with the working conditions and be unable to handle the stress at work and at home. Job hopping can be stressful, and changing positions may not be possible when the economy is poor.

SWITCHING TO PART-TIME WORK

Ideally, switching to part-time employment should not be a challenge. You may, however, want to consider working some from home to demonstrate your credibility and efficiency. As discussions continue, your track record of excellence could work in your favor.

Negotiate based on a specific project. If your current assignment requires skill sets that only you can provide, negotiate your time and availability accordingly. Demonstrate your flexibility by continuing on a full-time basis until the project is underway, then re-negotiate a part-time schedule in your favor.

If your goal is to work part time, consider the following:

- How many hours can you take off without affecting your benefits?
- Would your manager be supportive of the situation? If not, could you be more flexible?

WORK/LIFE BALANCE

We all have responsibilities, whether caring for children or elderly parents, or pursuing personal interests, activities, or hobbies. Workers must be equipped to resolve personal and workplace issues, juggle conflicting responsibilities, and balance personal and workplace roles.

At the same time, today's employers are constantly seeking ways to assist their workers in managing their job responsibilities and their personal responsibilities and needs. Strategies for work/life balance help create supportive, healthy work environments; strengthen employee commitment and loyalty; and result in more productive workplaces and improved customer satisfaction.

'We need to maintain a proper balance in our life by allocating the time we have. There are occasions where saying no is the best time management practice there is."

—Catherine Pulsife

As clinicians, we entered the field of nursing with a common goal—caring for, and about, others and providing the best possible outcomes. As professionals, we also have expectations from our work environment, from those with whom we work, and our future. Oprah Winfrey suggests that "right now you are one choice away from a new beginning—one that leads you toward becoming the fullest human being you can be."

If your path is paved with good intentions, but your work is unrewarding and your time is not your own, negotiate. Think things over and make a change.

Keeping Your Balance

FINDING FOCUS

For one day, notice how often you are not focusing on the task at hand. For example, during a phone call, are you thinking of what you have to do after you are done with the call? Are you straightening the clutter on your desk as you listen to a co-worker?

Before you make a call or keep an appointment, take a moment beforehand to say to yourself, "I will give this my full attention." Then do it.

TRACK YOUR TIME

Do you often find yourself at the end of the day wondering where the time went? Consider tracking how long it takes you to do routine tasks, so that you can better plan your time.

MAKE AN APPOINTMENT

Right now, make an appointment for lunch or another activity with a friend or relative you have been meaning to spend time with.

BECOME A NETWEAVER

Bob Littell coined the concept of NetWeaving, a form of networking that focuses on helping others instead of the "what's in it for me" concept of networking. Apply NetWeaving in your work and home life:

1. Take the time to make at least one connection between two people who can help each other, knowing that good deeds often reward the person doing them.

2. Identify one way you can share your expertise with others. It might be as simple as agreeing to share examples of reports you have written with someone who has never done one.

Source:
http://www.netweaving.com/articles/Part1-IntrotoNWing.pdf

"One cannot think well, love well, sleep well, if one has not dined well."

—Virginia Woolf

7

EAT, SLEEP, AND BE MERRY

Good nutrition, quality sleep, and a sense of fulfillment are essential ingredients for creating balance in one's life. As caregivers, we are stressed to the limit, and stress can challenge our well-being.

If your habits for nourishing and restoring yourself are not chosen consciously, chances are they may not actually be nourishing or restoring you. Any choice less than what is in your highest good is a choice that is going to deplete your storehouse of energy reserves and health; tax all the functions, organs, and cells of your body; and gradually impair wellness.

Sleep is one of the most significant factors in achieving mental and physical well-being. Second to sleep is adequate nutrition. Being "merry" as a result of quality sleep and wholesome nutrition is taught to us by babies and children. In observing the very young, we know that children become crankier, get sick more often, and are less fun to be with when they are hungry and experience inadequate, interrupted sleep.

In 2008, obesity was rated by parents as their number one health concern for their children (C.S. Mott Children's Hospital, 2007). The imbalances that are resulting in obesity, malnutrition, and sleep deprivation are contributing to the rise of other childhood and youth problems, all of which are of great concern. These include increasing high school drop-out rates, depression and teen suicide, drug usage (prescription, over the counter, and illicit drugs), violence, and an exponential increase in diseases and conditions such as anorexia, autism, attention deficit hyperactive disorder (ADHD), behavior disorders, and more.

NOTES ON NURSING

In the preface to *Notes on Nursing*, Florence Nightingale shares her philosophy and definition of nursing that have inspired nurses for decades. "Every day, the knowledge of nursing of how to put the constitution in such a state as that it will have no disease, or that it can recover from disease, takes a higher place. It is recognized as the knowledge which every one ought to have—distinct from medical knowledge, which only a professional can have."

"(When asked how to end world hunger, she replied:) 'Go home and feed your family.'"
—Mother Teresa

While the motto "moderation in all things" is a simple and helpful guideline to create health, it needs to be interwoven with another motto, "energy flows where attention goes." Balance in a human context refers to dispersing energy, time, and focus among the salient aspects of life in a manner that is satisfying and is congruent enough with those with whom life is shared.

Balance alone will not give us optimal health, for there is a continuum of health practices and choices that people can make no matter how balanced their life seems. For example, a person who has a stable life, with sufficient income, a stress-free job, supportive family and social relationships, and a sense of purpose could feel fairly balanced in his or her life despite a habit of smoking or drinking. The more people are able to come to balance or a harmonious relationship among the most important aspects of their lives, the more they will enjoy the energy for creating improved health, more satisfying lifestyle, and patterns that are more rewarding and generative. Balance or inner harmony will minimize stress and bring more joy in living, but it is not sufficient to generate high levels of health.

Moving along the continuum of optimal health requires increasing consciousness and awareness about lifestyle choices. Three areas in which increased awareness and choices can bring dramatic results are food choices, adequate sleep, and emotional resilience and competence.

The main themes of this chapter offer examples of "cultural blinders," realities to which society has become almost blinded. Simple suggestions point you in directions that will help you generate more balance and more health for yourself.

THE CULTURAL BLINDERS

I want to paint a picture of the elements of optimal health and of the capacity to live with vitality, radiance of heart, spirit, and joy. To do this, I'll offer examples of cultural blinders, and by doing so, it will help you think more outside the box and visualize a path for realizing success.

"A bird in the hand is the best way to eat chicken."

—Anonymous

Cultural blinders affect perception, thoughts, and behaviors by socializing people in what to focus on and what to avoid. In this, they share much with prejudices, but without the divisive and harmful judgmental attitude that is inherent in prejudice. Blinders are like lenses that distort our observations and experiences. What is seen, heard, or felt is barely registered because these elements are considered unimportant.

These blinders are present in every aspect of life. For example, with meal preference and preparation, few are aware of how severely compromised the nutritional value of the foods consumed today are, or how much sleep environments disturb capacities for deep sleep, so essential to health. Nor is much attention given to how worry, stress, anxiety, lack of vibrancy and joie de vivre decrease health and the capacity for making better choices. On the one hand, asking you to examine these aspects of your life is asking a lot. Changing nutritional and other health-care related habits is difficult, but I submit to you that your efforts to improve the quality of your health and your life will meet greater resistance the more you remain stuck in old habits that sabotage your well-being.

EAT

To examine your own blinders regarding eating and foods, take a mental walk through your local grocery store or supermarket. How much of what you find is fresh? How much is natural? How much is organic? Does the store tell you where the food comes from? It shouldn't take an E-coli in spinach or salmonella in tomatoes scare to convince you it's in your best interest to know how your food is grown, what is used to grow it, and where it comes from.

"One of the very nicest things about life is the way we must regularly stop whatever it is we are doing and devote our attention to eating."
—Luciano Pavarotti and William Wright

While it is outside the scope of this book to analyze scientific studies regarding food production and consumption, it is within our scope to recommend that you know what you are eating. Pick up any newspaper or watch the evening news and you will be told that diet and health are intimately connected. Unfortunately, most of what you read or hear points to one nutrient or another—the nutrient du jour, that miracle vitamin, mineral, or complex that the media pegs to be the newest cure-all. We encourage you to look at your food consumption from a holistic perspective, and not from a chemical or scientific perspective.

Educate yourself! The Johns Hopkins University has developed a Web site that serves as a repository and gateway to the intersection of public health and agriculture/food production. Called the Agriculture and Public Health Gateway (http://aphg.jhsph.edu/), it is a project of the Johns Hopkins Center for a Livable Future. Numerous Web sites address agriculture, running the gamut from industrial to small-scale farming and everything in between. Many other sites support and defend other aspects of food and health. However, the

Agriculture and Public Health Gateway provides a central place to access information about public health, agriculture, and the links between these two fields. A good place to start is by researching organic and sustainable foods. While you may not end up agreeing with the philosophies of these movements, you will get a complete picture of all the possible issues with industrial and chemical-intensive farming and can then research the alternative views.

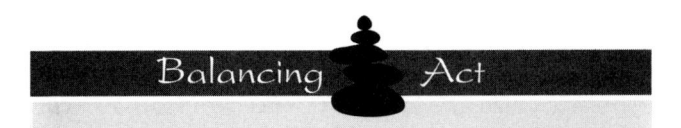

QUICK TIPS FOR SHOPPING HEALTHY

- Shop the perimeter of the grocery store, where fresh foods such as fruits, vegetables, dairy, meat, and fish are usually located.

- Avoid the center aisles where junk foods lurk. Choose "real" foods with as little processing and as few additives as possible. Remember, if you want more salt or sugar, you can always add it yourself.

- Avoid foods that contain more than five ingredients, artificial ingredients, or ingredients you can't pronounce.

Produce

The shorter the time between when produce is harvested and consumed, the higher the nutritional value of the food. Logically, this means you should buy produce from your local growers when the produce is in season. Local generally means within 150 miles of your home. We recommend visiting your farmers' markets—many towns and cities now have winter markets as well as spring, summer, and fall—and get to know the farmers. The more you learn about how the farmer farms, the better a consumer you can be. Another factor to consider when determining whether to purchase produce from a large retailer versus from your local farmers is food safety. While buying locally doesn't guarantee food safety, it does limit the processing, the time, the number of steps, and the number of human-to-food interactions between harvest and consumption.

"Shipping is a terrible thing to do to vegetables. They probably get jet-lagged, just like people."

—Elizabeth Berry

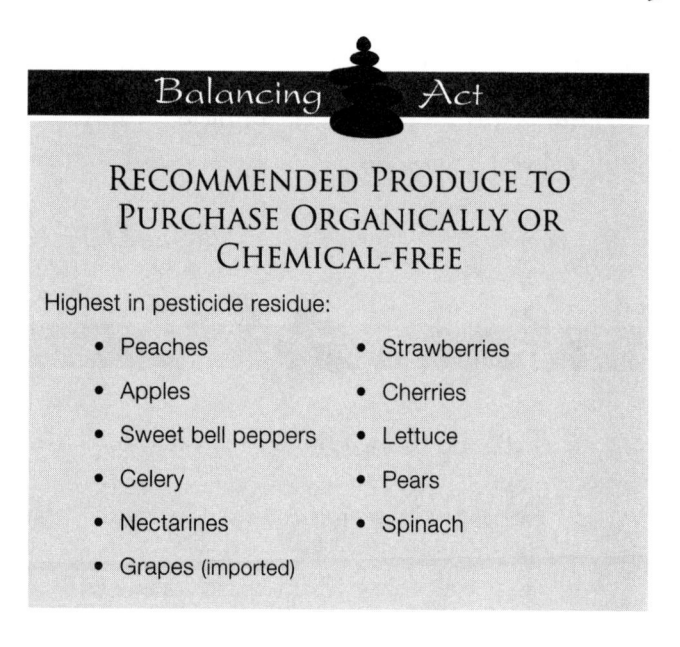

RECOMMENDED PRODUCE TO PURCHASE ORGANICALLY OR CHEMICAL-FREE

Highest in pesticide residue:

- Peaches
- Apples
- Sweet bell peppers
- Celery
- Nectarines
- Grapes (imported)
- Strawberries
- Cherries
- Lettuce
- Pears
- Spinach

Lowest in pesticide residue:

- Onions
- Avocado
- Sweet corn (frozen)
- Pineapples
- Mango
- Sweet peas (frozen)

- Asparagus
- Kiwi
- Bananas
- Cabbage
- Broccoli
- Eggplant

Source: Environmental Working Group

"If organic farming is the natural way, shouldn't organic produce just be called 'produce' and make the pesticide-laden stuff take the burden of an adjective?"

—Ymber Delecto

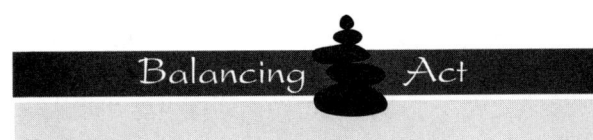

Balancing Act

TIPS FOR BUYING PRODUCE

1. Break your produce shopping down by season. You can find most produce items any time of year, but some are best during specific seasons.

2. In spring, buy apricots, artichokes, asparagus, avocados, beets, carrots, cauliflower, cherries, English peas, fava beans, radishes, rhubarb and spinach. It's best to ask a produce manager on the spot if something is worth buying. A

few tips: Avocados should be slightly soft and squeezable. Apricots should have a uniform color and shape and be slightly soft, as well. Spinach should have bright green, crisp leaves.

3. In summer, buy berries, corn, cucumbers, eggplant, figs, and garlic. Berries usually have a nice aroma when they're ripe. If they appear fresh on the underside of the container (not mushy or moldy), they're probably safe. Eggplants should be shiny and firm; the smaller they are means they're younger and sweeter. Figs are best when they're ripe and soft, almost shriveled.

4. In fall, buy apples, arugula, broccoli, Brussels sprouts, fennel, hard-shelled squash, pears, persimmons, pomegranate, sweet peppers and sweet potatoes. Broccoli shouldn't have any yellow spots, and should smell sweet—not like cabbage. Squash shouldn't have soft spots. Pears are best when firm but offering some give at the stem end.

6. Buy anytime if it looks safe. Out-of-season produce doesn't mean it's not still fresh and flavorful; it's probably just a bit smaller or has a weaker taste than in-season produce.

Source: eHow.com

Dairy

A synthetic growth hormone, recombinant Bovine Growth Hormone (rBGH) has been injected into U.S. dairy cows to artificially increase milk production since 1993 (Health Care Without Harm, n.d.). Both the American Nurses Association (ANA) and Physicians for Social Responsibility have issued policy statements against dairy products produced from cows injected with rBGH (American Nurses Association, 2008; Oregon Physicians for Social Responsibility, 2003). Both organizations specifically address the increase in disease rates in rBGH-injected cows and the potential for harm to humans, the increase in antibiotic use in rBGH-injected cows, which could lead to antibiotic resistance in humans, the potential cancer risk in humans through greater levels of insulin-like growth factor (IGF-1), and the fact that 30 countries to date have banned rBGH-injected dairy products.

"High-tech tomatoes. Mysterious milk. Supersquash. Are we supposed to eat this stuff? Or is it going to eat us?"

—Annita Manning

Meat

Most meats sold in large-scale grocery and big-box stores— beef, pork, chicken, and turkey—are raised on industrial/ factory farms that are sometimes referred to as confinement animal feeding operations (CAFOs). CAFOs are agricultural facilities that house and feed a large number of animals in a confined area for 45 days or more during any 12-month period. These are factory farms that practice raising farm animals in high-density populations to optimize profit. Confinement practices create situations that can be conducive to disease and lameness (Union of Concerned Scientists, 2006). Thus, most animals in CAFOs and other factory farms are prophylactically fed antibiotics to promote quick growth and to compensate for crowded, stressful, unsanitary conditions. Some CAFOs also supply tranquilizing drugs in the feed or water to keep the stressed animals calmer and to prevent potential injuries.

"The way you cut your meat reflects the way you live."

—Confucius

The Centers for Disease Control (CDC) have a statement posted on their Web site addressing CAFOs:

Public Health Concerns

People who work with livestock may develop adverse health effects, including chronic and acute respiratory illnesses and musculoskeletal injuries, and may be exposed to infections that travel from animals to humans. Residents in areas surrounding CAFOs report nuisances, such as odor and flies. In studies of CAFOs, CDC has shown that chemical and infectious compounds from swine and poultry waste are able to migrate into soil and water near CAFOs. Scientists do not yet know whether or how the migration of these compounds affects human health.

Pollutants possibly associated with manure-related discharges at CAFOs include:

Antibiotics, which may contribute to the development of antibiotic-resistant pathogens

Pathogens, such as parasites, bacteria, and viruses, which can cause disease in animals and humans

Nutrients, such as ammonia, nitrogen, and phosphorus, which can reduce oxygen in surface waters, encourage the growth of harmful

algal blooms, and contaminate drinking-water
sources

Pesticides and hormones, which researchers
have associated with hormone-related changes
in fish

Solids, such as feed and feathers, which can
limit the growth of desirable aquatic plants in
surface waters and protect disease-causing mi-
croorganisms

Trace elements, such as arsenic and copper,
which can contaminate surface waters and possibly harm human health

Researchers do not yet know whether or how
these or other substances from CAFOs may affect human health. Therefore, CDC supports
efforts to address these questions.

For many health care professionals, there is a significant concern that overuse of antibiotics in the food chain is contributing
to antibiotic-resistant bacteria strains in animals and humans.
Both the American Nurses Association and the American Medical Association are opposed to the non-medically indicated routine dosing of antibiotics to livestock. Organizations lobbying
for laws abolishing this practice are Keep Antibiotics Working
(http://www.keepantibioticsworking.org/new/index.cfm) and
the Alliance for the Prudent Use of Antibiotics (http://www.
tufts.edu/med/apua/). As healthcare providers and as consum-
ers, we should be aware of the issues and make informed decisions for ourselves and our patients/clients regarding consuming meat products from CAFO animals.

Shopping

Where do you go to find simple, healthy foods? Check out fresh markets. You walk in and smell the aroma of fresh vegetables and fruit; your eyes are flooded with beautiful arrays of colorful, fresh vegetables and fruits filling the space. In addition to local and farmers' markets, investigate ethnic markets. You will find a wide selection of foods, with few to no processed or highly refined products.

Mentally go through your pantry and refrigerator at home. How often do you stop to examine your assumptions about the foods you are buying?

Convenience Foods

Most of us today were raised with convenience foods. It has become our habit to rely on convenient, processed, prepared food. Hectic work schedules lead to overuse of convenience and fast food. Eating while driving a vehicle or on a cell phone, at the workstation, and during stressful business meals detracts from our balance and makes digestion difficult. Make a point of setting aside time to eat. Even if you cannot get away from fast food immediately, make yourself make time to eat at a table, not at your desk or in your car. It's a first step, but an important one. Set a goal for weaning yourself off fast food. If you need motivation to get off fast food, read *Fast Food Nation* by Eric Schlosser or rent *Super Size Me*, a documentary by Morgan Spurlock. There is little that is redeemable from a nutritional standpoint about fast food. For microwavable foods, read the labels. Don't buy anything with more than five ingredients or that has ingredients you cannot pronounce or do not know what they are.

"Sugar is a type of bodily fuel, yes, but your body runs about as well on it as a car would."

—V.L. Allineare

Eating Out

As overextended professionals, we are more likely to eat to try to increase our energy. At these times, we typically choose foods that spike our insulin levels. They also tend to be ones that are easiest to get into our mouths quickly and on the go. The easiest are too often the worst for us: highly refined, processed, and packaged foods. Most restaurants will cater to special dietary requests. Never hesitate to ask for healthful choices. And, if you choose to eat organically, ask chefs about the sources of their food. They are more likely to buy from local and sustainable sources if customers ask. If you aren't comfortable asking, then seek out restaurants in your community that are already committed to organic or sustainable foods. Frequently, these restaurants have the best chefs as they are the most particular about their ingredients.

Balancing Act

GOOD, GOOD, GOOD, GOOD DIGESTION

1. **Chew until liquid.** By chewing foods until liquid, two things are accomplished: First, tremendous burden is taken off the stomach and intestines, allowing for more energy to be available for healing, repair, and maintenance of

tissues and organs. Second, chewing foods until liquid allows powerful digestive enzymes in saliva to thoroughly mix with food, an essential first step for optimal digestion.

2. **Minimize drinking water and other fluids while eating.** Drinking water and other fluids can cause dilution of stomach acids and digestive enzymes, making them less effective at breaking down food. Whenever possible, it is best to drink fluids before and 2 hours after meals. Reducing the amount of salt and spices added to foods is helpful in reducing the need to drink fluids with meals.

3. **Avoid physical exertion following meals.** Approximately one-half of the body's entire blood supply is needed by the digestive organs following a meal. Physical exertion diverts blood away from our digestive organs, thereby reducing the efficiency of our digestive processes. Taking time to physically rest for approximately 1 hour following meals will allow for adequate blood supply to the digestive organs and optimal digestion.

Source: http://drbenkim.com/

Eating In

Can you remember when the family meal was a time where all family members were together, engaging in a ritual that brought cohesion, relaxation, good conversation, and laughter—all great elements for proper digestion? Can you bring back the aroma of home-cooked foods, memories of special tablecloths, the best dishes, and the fun of a candlelight dinner? Perhaps you had the bounty of coming from a family where everyone pitched in to help with the preparation and clean-up, so that when the meal was over, everyone could sit down and relax for the rest of the evening. Perhaps you didn't, but you can definitely create your own rituals, traditions, and lasting memories now.

"After dinner sit a while, and after supper walk a mile."

—English saying

The Slow Food movement (www.slowfoodusa.org) is a call to reverse trends that have taken people away from the meal as a family and community ritual. The Slow Food movement—living the slow life—is about pleasure and taste, knowledge and choice. Once we begin to take an interest in the enjoyment of food, and in finding out where our food comes from, we can begin to see the effects of these choices. When we shorten the distance—both literally and figuratively—that our food travels to get to us, we are participating in the Slow Food movement. Slow Food is about coming together as a food community—community producers and co-producers come together at the farm, in the market, and at the table to create and enjoy food that is good, clean, and fair.

Nutrients

Even if you eat only the best foods, follow optimal digestion practices, exercise, and take care of yourself in other ways, you may still need nutrient supplementation to achieve increased energy and health. Additionally, attending to the pH balance in our bodies by drinking properly alkinalized and filtered water and eating a higher ratio of alkaline to acid-producing foods is critical for optimal cellular metabolism. Balancing pH levels and improving the intracellular transport of nutrients and water aid in the prevention of autoimmune and other chronic diseases. Additionally, individuals vary in metabolic rate and genetic predisposition. People can be eating foods that are considered good and healthy, but these foods may not be good for them. The more people eat according to the specific needs of their bodies, the healthier they will continue to be and the younger they will feel and look. Consider consulting with a nutritionist or holistic practitioner to ascertain your nutrient, pH, hormone, and enzyme levels to determine the best supplementation for you.

SLEEP

Cellular metabolism and utilization of the nutrients consumed require the proper quality sleep. The two are synergistic and enhance each other. As a culture, we are experiencing a dramatic increase in sleep deprivation and disturbances.

"Laugh and the world laughs with you, snore and you sleep alone."

—Anthony Burgess

Most bedrooms now have TVs, sound systems, computers, phones, and alarm clocks. They are no longer just a place for sleep. This is true of even children's rooms. Unfortunately, these units emit electromagnetic frequencies (EMGs) that are disruptive to the human energy system. Many people fear the dark, so they choose to sleep with nightlights on or to fall asleep with the TV on. In addition, bedrooms can often become the catch-all for an overabundance of stuff that we do not want to leave out in the public areas of our homes. Whether books, magazines, papers, or clothes, the more our bedrooms become filled and busy, the poorer the air quality becomes.

Patterns of late-night activity, or lack of it, also are powerful contributors to sleep disturbances. Though many are in denial about this, watching media where intense human drama, violence, and action are blasted out in rapid-fire images can be dizzying, affecting us energetically and emotionally. Pushing our bodies into the sympathetic nervous system, when we should be gearing down within the parasympathetic system of slowed respirations, heart rate activity, and digestion, prevents the relaxed state necessary for quality sleep. Swing shifts, night shifts, long shifts, and deadlines of all kinds are prescriptions for sleep difficulties.

"Fatigue is the best pillow."

—Benjamin Franklin

As children, we have resilience to these kinds of energy depletions, so it seems not to affect us then, but as we continue to deplete energy through unhealthy practices, the deficiencies become increasingly apparent. That being said, it is also true that an increasing number of children experience more problems sleeping. Perhaps their resilience is being negatively affected even earlier by the combination of poor eating habits, living in a stressed family, having expectations for their performance that are too demanding, not having sufficiently healthy social interactions, being too sedentary, and more.

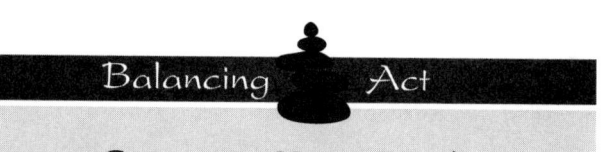

CATCHING YOUR ZZZZ'S

Ask yourself, "What are the behaviors and conditions in my life that might be reducing the quality of my sleep? In what ways have I been blinded by the choices I have made regarding my sleep?"

Some simple tips to help your sleep:

* If you're not ready to ban the TV, sound system, and other energy emitters from your bedroom, keep them on a power strip and turn off the power strip when you go to bed. This will minimize the energy output while you sleep.

* Don't eat within 2 hours of sleeping. Your organs need to be restoring themselves while you sleep, not trying to digest food.

* Don't drink caffeinated beverages past late afternoon.

* De-clutter your bedroom to create a feeling of peace and harmony.

* Do deep breathing exercises before going to bed.

* Once in bed, try to empty your mind. If you are concentrating on or worrying about falling asleep, you won't.

Adults are sleep deprived by as much as 1 to 1 1/2 hours per night. As health care professionals, we are much more aware of some of the horrific effects of prolonged sleep deprivation, but we ourselves frequently fall into the same trap. Sleep deprivation affects judgment, memory and concentration, emotions, speech, and thought processes, and often affects hormonal changes that increase weight gain.

"Sleeping is no mean art: for its sake one must stay awake all day."

—Friedrich Nietzsche

For those who work in hospitals, there are additional challenges. Nurses are often required to work double shifts if there is no staffing replacement, sometimes leaving at 1 a.m. to return at 7 a.m. the next day. We have become experts at prescribing and providing optimal care to our client population, yet how many times over the years have we provided a similar standard of care for ourselves? How many of us felt that we could catch a 3-hour catnap before leaving for our next "tour of duty"? If we thought to pack a lunch, it is often consumed while driving or at the nurses' station or in the linen room. We dehydrate ourselves by not taking the time to drink sufficient water, and then dehydrate ourselves more by drinking coffee to stay awake. It is no wonder that when a working parent collapses onto the sofa to spend time reading a favorite bedtime story to a child, the parent falls asleep before the story ends.

It is ironic that health care professionals are often compelled to work in systems that are strangely not designed to support our own health. Sleep deprivation then becomes a powerful contributor to professional burnout and compassion fatigue, both of which health care providers are at risk of developing.

When was the last time that you relived a favorite bedtime routine from your past? Do you remember the special feeling and aroma of a warm bath, clean pajamas, and freshly laundered sheets with a relaxing bedtime story and a cup of warm milk or bedtime tea?

"A good laugh and a long sleep are the best cures in the doctor's book."

—Irish Proverb

When was the most recent time that you awakened refreshed, full of energy, and ready to take on the challenges of a new day? Quality sleep is absolutely essential for physical and emotional well-being. Deep sleep without waking in the night (which decreases the amount of time spent in deep sleep and in the rapid eye movement [REM] cycles) is necessary for body repair and restoration, immune system support, and coping with stress. The depth of the sleep, firmness and quality of the mattress, proper body alignment, and proper temperature are important variables in providing quality sleep.

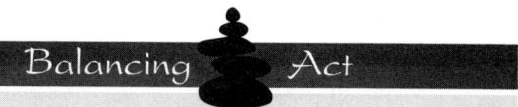

Balancing Act

MATTRESS MATTERS

Americans spend one-third of their lives sleeping, so it makes sense to invest in a sleep set that can improve your comfort and overall health. These tips are good to consider when selecting a mattress:

- **Shop for Support.** Look for a mattress that provides uniform support from head to toe; if there are gaps between your body and the mattress (such as at the waist), you're not getting the full support you need. Mattresses can be too firm; pay close attention to uncomfortable pressure on prominent body features such as the shoulders, hips, and low back. Because your body is pressing down on the springs at the low areas, these springs push back, creating pressure points. A pressure point can create the same effect as when you compress an injury to stop bleeding. That is, it restricts blood flow to these areas.

- **Shop for Comfort.** When mattress shopping, give each option a good trial run before you buy; lie down on a mattress for a minimum of 5 to 10 minutes to get a good idea of its comfort level. If you cannot find a comfortable position, you probably have the wrong mattress.

- **Shop for Size.** Does the bed provide enough room for both you and your sleeping partner, if you have one, to stretch and roll over? The ideal mattress will also minimize the transfer of movement from one sleeping partner to the other, which means one person shouldn't feel motion as the other leaves the bed.

Source: American Chiropractic Association.

Additionally, there are a number of specialized mattresses to consider:

- **Magnetic Mattress.** The earth produces a magnetic field that reaches from one pole to the other. Throughout history, human beings spent their waking and sleeping hours exposed to this magnetic field. City and suburban structures and electrical and microwave towers reduce or interfere with exposure to this natural and grounding magnetic field. A magnetic mattress cocoons the body, returning you to your natural state of balance and enhancing the sleep process.

- **Organic Mattress.** Many modern mattresses contain toxic chemicals used in the construction process that outgas and can harm our health and impede sleep. Organic mattresses use only organic materials without harmful chemicals.

- **Far-Infrared Technology.** Far-infrared energy is part of all living things. It is constantly absorbing energy and reflecting it as gentle warmth. Far-infrared absorbs moisture, reflects heat, and insulates the body. The technology offers all-season comfort.

- **Rubberthane Technology.** A natural way to relieve stress and discomfort is with massage. Several sleep products attempt to reproduce this sensation with a textured or raised egg-carton-like surface similar to the 3/4″ egg-crate overlay used in the past. Every time that you move during sleep, the Rubberthane nodules help to ease tension and relax the body.

BE MERRY

For those of us who devote our professional lives to helping others who are sick, suffering, and struggling, there are certain caveats and pitfalls in addition to the general issue of professionals overextending themselves.

"Even if happiness forgets you a little bit, never completely forget about it."

—Jacques Prévert

As compassionate and empathetic people, we can pick up the emotions and energy of those with whom we are working. Despite our empathy, often we are not sensitive enough about ourselves to realize how much we do pick up and how this can affect our moods, our energy, and our general outlook on life.

Emotionally, most people will distract themselves from negative feelings, take them out on others or themselves, or shut down their emotional selves. Very few people have the awareness to shift out of negative emotions and beliefs, brighten their perspectives, and make more positive choices by actually releasing the negativity they are experiencing.

Indeed, Eckhart Tolle, in his book *The Power of Now*, asks the reader to consider the ramifications of this scenario: Imagine that everyone who was on antidepressants or anxiolitics, and who used alcohol or drugs, suddenly had no access to such mood- and mind-altering substances. Engaging in this imagery gives a powerful indication of just how out of balance we are.

A state of vibrant health is our birthright. At our core level, we are vibrant, alive, positive, and happy. But sadly, life's experiences and the stress of daily existence cause our bodies to degenerate, our emotions to go absent without leave (AWOL), and our souls to feel disconnected.

"The best way to cheer yourself up is to try to cheer somebody else up."

—Mark Twain

Despite the medical, lifestyle, and nutritional advances that contribute to greater health and the possibility of longer and healthier lives, we appear to be becoming less healthy. It has been suggested that in the Unites States, this generation of children will be the first in many generations not to live as long as their parents, mainly due to lifestyle choices. Our concepts of what it means to get old have everything to do with choices we make now about our health. The sleep we get and the nutrition we provide ourselves with are two of the four most important healthy lifestyle elements, the others being exercise and social support.

This has major implications for mood. Being merry is not easy to pull off for most of us who experience stress. Stress comes in many sizes, from periodic stressful situations and deadlines to prolonged, seemingly intractable stressful dynamics; to health problems; and to stress reactions from earlier and unhealed traumas in our lives. And with each of these kinds of stress, the level of stress experienced can run the full range from minimal to catastrophic. Stress is a key risk factor in all disease conditions, impacting the delicate balance of body, mind, and spirit.

"There is no cosmetic for beauty like happiness."

—Lady Blessington

Once you have more energy, it is much easier to make whatever changes you want to make. With more vitality, you participate more fully in other aspects of your life, are more able to attend to projects that have been building up, and begin to feel immediately better about yourself for accomplishing more and feeling more on top of your own life.

Emotional energy is the most important and vital energy we have. Having sufficient emotional energy is the result of learning to harmonize the needs, involvements, and choices that we make, while sustaining sufficiently healthy lifestyles, so that our bodies can generate the physical energy necessary to feel good. Emotional energy then is the barometer of being balanced and healthy enough for living with vitality, enthusiasm, connection, fulfillment, and inner peace.

Without it, the stresses of daily life take a greater toll, but with it, a number of things happen energetically that have profound effects on satisfaction and sense of fulfillment in the world. Others are drawn to those with sufficient emotional energy, more opportunities seem to present themselves, and the interactions are more positive, generating energy rather than absorbing it through negative dynamics and experiences.

"Happiness is like a butterfly which, when pursued, is always beyond our grasp, but, if you will sit down quietly, may alight upon you."

—Nathaniel Hawthorne

According to Mira Kirshenbaum, you are suffering from emotional fatigue if you are feeling irritable or intruded upon, are easily annoyed, have difficulty coping, and are not doing what you really need to be doing to be fully functioning in your life. Other signs of emotional fatigue are when your heart isn't in the things you are doing, and it has been more than a week since you allowed yourself to do something of real enjoyment. It always takes more energy to make changes. Sometimes we have the extra energy; it is just a matter of strengthening our will sufficiently to add new, healthier behaviors or to stop counterproductive ones. But, if we are pushing ourselves too hard, it is much more difficult to generate the energy required to make a change.

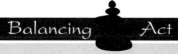

Balancing Act

RECHARGE YOUR BATTERIES

Here are suggestions for increasing your energy, especially useful for those who are depressed and whose energy is depleted.

- Take 3 1/2 tablespoons of organic coconut oil daily to increase your energy. Spread the dose throughout the day.

- Drink barley grass. Due to its detoxifying properties, begin with a low dose and gradually increase to the recommended dose to avoid side effects such as fatigue and increased bowel activity. Be sure to drink plenty of water to facilitate detoxification.

- Add high-quality magnetic insoles to your shoes.

- Go to bed earlier. Some believe that the earlier you retire, the better sleep you get. Even 1 hour earlier at night can make a noticeable difference the next morning. You may awaken feeling more refreshed and ready for the day. If you are already getting sufficient rest, the earlier sleep will provide extra energy, and since you'll probably awaken earlier, too, an early session of yoga, meditation, or prayer becomes more possible.

- Upon awakening, jot down all the early morning thoughts you have that you don't want to forget, then grab the mat for yoga or stretching to get the lymphatic system moving, stretch the muscles, and increase physical flexibility. This translates into more emotional and mental flexibility, perhaps even more creativity as you go through your day.

- Julia Cameron suggests "morning pages" for those who awaken with worries. Quickly write them all down, and you have done something to release them, making it easier to get on with your day.

Taking prescription medications for depression and anxiety often helps people feel better and can sometimes be life-saving. But prescription medications are often prescribed without enough information about possible health risks, both in adjusting to the drug and in potential short- and long-term side effects. Too few doctors and patients know enough about alternatives to drugs to decrease or eliminate depressive and anxious symptoms. From the perspective of creating more inner balance, there are many methods, supplements, activities, and therapies that may eliminate the symptoms and help the person create more health—something the anti-depressants and anxiolitics won't do.

"The best vitamin to be a happy person is B1."

—Author Unknown

Sleep may be a challenge, especially in those working multiple shifts and irregular hours. Alternatives to sleep medication may include homeopathic blends, flower essences, and essential oils, all of which relax the body and mind, creating a good internal environment for restful sleep. Taking calcium and magnesium before bed, melatonin (unless contraindicated due to certain types of depression), valerian root extracts or teas, and kava kava are all excellent ways for promoting better sleep and thus better mental health. Also consider seeing a chiropractor who specializes in glandular/hormonal balancing. Hormonal and glandular health is important to overall emotional/mental health. Remember, it is during rapid eye movement (REM) sleep that memory is restored and cellular health is enhanced.

Keeping Your Balance

Take this simple self-awareness test and eat, sleep, and be merry ... from this point forward.

We invite you now to rate your own levels of well-being and health. On a scale from 0-10, where 10 represents the best possible it seems that one could feel (not necessarily you, since you might have the tendency to deflate how good you could feel), how would you rate yourself on each of the following questions?

What is the worst you have ever felt emotionally?

What is the worst you have ever felt physically/ energetically?

What is the healthiest you have ever felt?

What is the happiest you have ever felt?

How good (combining both health and happiness or well-being) would you like to feel?

How good do you believe you can feel?

How good (physically, emotionally, and energetically) are you feeling now?

How balanced do you feel (both internal health, including mental, emotional, physical, spiritual, and social aspects, and being in the world elements of work, family, friends, and self time)?

Answering these questions gives you both a base line and a road map for yourself as you continue to improve your overall state of well-being. Use these numbers to track your efforts and your experience daily. You could also use this to track how well you ate, how well you slept, how much energy you have, how bright your mood is. Tracking how often and what kind of exercise you do, and what kind of centering/grounding you do (meditation, prayer, etc.) is an excellent way to increase your awareness of how much your lifestyle choices affect your well-being and how well you are really feeling.

"What soap is to the body, laughter is to the soul."

−Yiddish Proverb

8

LAUGHTER: THE BEST MEDICINE

Without question, one of the best feelings in the world is being overcome with uncontrollable laughter. You know the kind, when you laugh so hard you cry, and you keep chuckling each time you relive the moment, even hours after the fit of laughter has left you. Laughing, it turns out, lowers blood pressure, reduces stress hormones, increases muscle flexibility, and boosts the immune function (Berk et al., 1989). It does this by raising the levels of infection-fighting proteins and cells that produce disease-destroying antibodies—T-cells and antibodies IgA and IgB. Additionally, one study at the University of Maryland Medical Center revealed a connection between laughter and the healthy functioning of blood vessels (Miller, 2000).

With today's hectic pace, we need a few moments of daily laughter—the more the better. It is free of charge and readily available. In the face of frequently dispiriting news from around the globe, it is easy to become glum and irritable, and that can quickly and quietly throw off your balance.

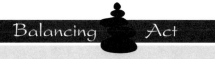

Balancing Act

HUMOR THROUGHOUT HISTORY

Biblical Times
Book of Proverbs 17:22: "A cheerful heart does good like a medicine, but a broken spirit makes one sick."

14th Century
French surgeon Henri de Mondeville used humor therapy to enhance surgical recovery. He wrote, "Let the surgeon take care to regulate the whole regimen of the patient's life for joy and happiness, allowing his relatives and special friends to cheer him and by having someone tell him jokes."

16th Century:
Robert Burton, an English parson and scholar, used humor to cure melancholy.

Martin Luther used humor therapy for pastoral counseling.

17th Century
Herbert Spencer, sociologist, used humor to relieve tension.

18th Century
Immanuel Kant used humor to restore equilibrium.

William Battle used humor to treat the sick.

20th Century
Clowns were brought into U.S. hospitals to cheer children afflicted with polio.

The Gesundheit Institute was founded by Patch Adams (1972).

Norman Cousins published his book, *Anatomy of an Illness as Perceived by the Patient* (1979), based on his own experiences using humor to recover from ankylosing spondylitis.

Release of "Patch Adams" film starring Robin Williams (1998).

21st Century

Laugh out loud (lol) therapy becomes a part of our daily lives through text messaging, e-mailing, instant messaging, and other forms of electronic communication.

Adapted from Laughter Therapy (http://www.freewebs. com/laughtertherapy/humourtherapy.htm).

PHYSIOLOGY OF LAUGHTER

Laughter is a combination of modified respiratory movements: inspiration followed by many short convulsive expirations, during which the rima glottidis—the opening between the true vocal cords and the arytenoid cartilages—remains open and the vocal folds vibrate. Laughter is accompanied by characteristic rhythms of movement and facial expressions. Patients who can smile benefit from relaxed muscles, released neuropeptides, and vasodilated blood vessels.

Laughter is therapeutic because it relaxes us and gives us a better perspective: A period of laughter gives us the opportunity to look at things differently and defuses painful emotions.

The American Holistic Nurses Association, in its *Core Curriculum for Holistic Nursing* (1997), addresses the physiologic benefits of humor and laughter and calls laughter a wonderful tonic for the body. The core principles include:

- Humor as a cognitive skill that uses both sides of the brain.
- Laughter as an antidote to stress.
- Laughter as a way to increase the number of helper T cells (Berk et al., 1989).

PSYCHOLOGY AND SOCIOLOGY OF LAUGHTER

Laughter is a universal, non-language-specific human phenomenon. The primary reason for laughter appears to be to bring people together (Provine, 2000). Indeed, laughter may well be the first verbal form of communication among humans and other primate species (Provine, 2004). Jo-Anne Bachorowski, PhD, a psychology professor at Vanderbilt University, has begun to expand on Provine's work. We use laughter, she posits, to elicit positive reactions from other people and to communicate to them that we mean them no harm (2001). According to Provine (2004), laughter almost never occurs in solitary situations and is a contagious phenomenon.

The range of laughter-arousing experiences is enormous, from physical tickling to mental titillations. Yet it is an intellectual and emotional process enabling us to relieve pent-up emotions. "After all, with even the most intellectual brands of humor, laughter is ultimately an expression of emotion—joy, surprise, nervousness, amusement" (Doskoch, 1996, ¶6).

HEALTH BENEFITS

Laughter has enormous health benefits for those with diverse clinical conditions from chronic diseases, such as diabetes; for lowering risks of heart attacks; and for everything in between. In the world in which we live, replete with modern medical breakthroughs, who would ever dream that something as simple as laughter could induce such amazing benefits for your health?

A study of patients with type 2 diabetes revealed that laughter helps regulate gene expression (Hayashi et al., 2006). Studies also suggest that laughter positively affects rheumatoid arthritis by affecting the level of the condition as well as providing psychological benefits in controlling stress and stress-related conditions (Matsuzaki et al., 2006). Laughter may even protect people against a heart attack (Miller, 2000).

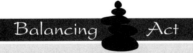

Balancing Act

WATCH AND LAUGH

Life can sometimes be serious and tiring, but if you look around and can draw some laughter out of what may seem mundane, you could possibly be helping your health. The writer/editor Norman Cousins claimed to have resolved a diagnosis of ankylosing spondylitis by watching Laurel and Hardy and Marx Brothers movies. In his book, *Anatomy of an Illness as Perceived by the Patient,* Cousins chronicles the way in which he laughed his way to health. He wrote that 10 minutes of genuine belly laughter had an anesthetic effect on his pain that, in turn, granted him at least 2 hours of pain-free sleep. When the pain-killing effect of the laughter wore off, he would start the process all over again by turning on another movie (Cousins, 1979).

> The next time you need to laugh, consider getting out your favorite comedies and let the good times roll!

Laughter makes it easier to handle life and its challenges, because it puts us "in the moment." When we are in the moment, we are less aware of our problems. Remember a time when you have laughed and things have somehow seemed different. Going back to childhood, our parents and grandparents would try to get us to laugh through our tears after a skinned knee. Later, it was over a broken heart or a betrayed friendship. Throughout life, even at the lowest points, such as the death of a close loved one, remembered laughter can lighten the load and help restore equilibrium to our lives. Laughter is therapeutic because it relaxes us and gives us a better perspective: A period of laughter gives us the opportunity to look at things differently and defuses painful emotions. With practice, we can and should make laughter a part of our everyday lives.

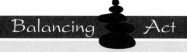

Balancing Act

THE CEDARS-SINAI EXPERIENCE

At the 2007 Annual Meeting of the American Psychiatric Association in San Diego, California, researchers from Cedars-Sinai Medical Center showcased a study on brain tumors and laughter. The researchers investigated the dispositions toward humor of a group of depressed patients in the outpatient psychiatric department at Cedars-Sinai. Patients were asked to complete a short questionnaire comprised of a regular depression scale as well as Svebak's Sense of Humor Questionnaire. Svebak, a professor at the Norwegian University of Science and

Technology (NTNU), has examined the relationship between humor and health for years.

In the Cedars-Sinai presentation, the authors shared the following benefits from laughter:

- Reduced cortisol levels in the body

- Improved circulation

- Stimulated nervous system

- Improved immune functioning

- Stronger heart

- Lower blood pressure

- Release of endorphins

And, they suggested the following laughter modalities:

- Subscribe to e-mail newsletters that provide daily jokes.

- Watch a comedy two or three times per weekend.

- See a live comedian or watch one on television.

- Wave to yourself in the mirror.

Do a silly, nonconforming thing each and every day.

LEARNING TO LAUGH

We can easily incorporate humor into our work lives. We may not all be comedians and clowns, but we can all bring light-heartedness and joy into our work. Use these helpful hints:

In office-work environments:

- Decorate your office with toys that you and your visitors can play with when things get difficult. Play dough is a great office tool!
- Start a Laugh-In club with contests for the best (appropriate) jokes or clowning around.
- Make those around you laugh at least three times a day, and they will return the favor.
- Keep silly photos of you and your loved ones around you.
- Keep "dress up" items such as silly costumes found at garage or yard sales in your office. When the stress gets too high, walking the halls in a curly rainbow wig or Superman cape can lighten the atmosphere considerably.
- Bring in music that calms you.
- Keep a basket of stress-relievers.

In patient-care environments:

- Determine to do your best to help each of your patients laugh several times during your shift. They will likely return the favor, and you will in turn feel better.
- Keep toys available to share with your co-workers and patients.
- Throw patient parties for no reason.
- Encourage appropriate playfulness that doesn't endanger anyone.
- Learn to draw caricatures and share them with your patients and co-workers.
- Consider a laughter team that visits patient-care areas and shares stories.

"If you can laugh at something, it ceases to be so overwhelming."

A good example of humor in the patient-care area is when a patient complains about the coverage provided by their hospital gown, we could respond with: "The doctor did admit you for observation," or, following a procedure, you might say, "You look great on paper—how do you feel?"

When beginning work in a new area, familiarizing yourself with a new team of professionals and environment can be a challenge. So, too, is a new patient workload. A single attempt at humor by pretending to not be able to find a patient's heartbeat or pretending to find Mickey Mouse in a child's ears quickly crosses barriers and establishes a good relationship.

Don't forget humor in your personal life too. Remember, a smile goes a long way, and laughter will:

- Promote a positive environment.
- Create an air of trust.
- Cheer you and others around you.
- Rechannel energy to something more positive.
- Release tension.
- Reduce stress.
- Work the diaphragm and increase the body's ability to use oxygen.

If you can laugh at something, it ceases to be so overwhelming. Remember: Laughter is contagious. Have something in your workplace that automatically makes you smile. Once you're smiling, spread it around and make your co-workers and patients smile too!

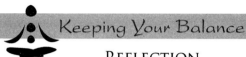

Keeping Your Balance

REFLECTION

What are two things you can do tomorrow to bring humor into your workplace and your home?

LAUGHTER AND HAPPINESS

Laughter and happiness go hand in hand. Learn more about authentic happiness:
http://www.authentichappiness.sas.upenn.edu/Default.aspx

Consider joining or starting a laughter club:
http://www.worldlaughtertour.com

"Dream lofty dreams, and as you dream, so shall you become. Your vision is the promise of what shall one day be."

—James Allen

9

DREAM BIG

Today, somewhere, someone is going to go back to school to improve his or her life. Someone is going to look in the mirror and see a need to lose a little weight, and that will spur the decision to become healthy. Someone will run a first marathon. Someone, somewhere, is going to set out on a pathway to success and reach beyond dreams to change lives.

Often, we dream big dreams and have great aspirations. These are waking dreams, planned-for dreams—the kind of dreams sometimes referred to as ambition. We all know the names of many successful dreamers—those whose actions made their dreams come true—because we see them frequently in the media. Among them are:

- Barack Obama, first African-American elected president of the United States.
- Michael Phelps, winner of 14 Olympic gold medals, the most by any Olympian in history.
- Shannon Miller, the only American to rank among the top 10 all-time gymnasts, and, the only female athlete to be inducted into the U.S. Olympic Hall of Fame, twice! (Individual in 2006 and Team in 2008.)

- Oprah Winfrey, internationally syndicated talk-show host and media mogul who is ranked among the most powerful people in history.
- Yao Ming, the first Chinese National Basketball Association (NBA) star.
- J.K. Rowling, writer of the Harry Potter book series, which has sold more than 400 million copies worldwide, been translated into 65+ languages, and credited with inspiring many adolescents and young adults to turn off their televisions and pick up books instead.
- Tiger Woods, a professional golfer and one of the most successful athletes in history.
- Bill Gates, founder of Microsoft and billionaire philanthropist.

This list could go on and on. We all have heroes or heroines who inspire and motivate us, and not all of them make the evening news or even their local, weekly newspapers. These people are no less successful as dreamers because they haven't become the president of the United States or won 14 Olympic gold medals. What makes someone a dreamer is the ability to envision a possibility for the future and then make that vision a reality, one step at a time.

Balancing Act

WHO ARE YOUR DREAMERS?

Martin Luther King's famous speech, "I Have a Dream," has been changing people's lives across America and the world ever since he uttered those four powerful words.

And, although his life came to an early, tragic end, his family and his followers kept his dream alive.

Within the health care arena, we are often called upon to build coalitions; it is an integral part of the survival process. Wendy Kopp, founder and president of Teach for America, is a coalition builder and someone from whom we can learn. Her highly developed leadership skills and use of social strategies led to the creation of a privately funded, nonprofit organization with 15 offices. Kopp transformed the public education system at three levels: state policy, district teaching, and national public awareness. Kopp, formerly a "doer" herself, has grown tremendously, empowering others along the way. She, like Dr. King, had a dream. She made this dream a reality. In the process, Teach for America Inc., became a holding company for three other programs—Teach, Learning Project, and Teach for America—that are changing the lives of people across the United States.

Think about your dreamers, those who have risen through the ranks and achieved great things. Write their names and their success stories.

Next, create your own dream inventory. Dreams may be good or bad. Many people share universal dreams. Some of these may include:

- Falling in front of a car or train.

- Suffering natural disasters.

- Flying in a plane.

- Appearing naked in public.

- Losing your teeth.

- Finding or losing money.

You may have experienced some of these as a child, and you may have wondered what they meant. This list includes a number of threatening dreams—you may consider them nightmares. A good way to deal with them is to reverse them—make them positive things that happen to you, like:

- Saving someone from falling in front of a car or train.

- Surviving a natural disaster and saving others.

- Piloting a plane to a safe landing.

You get the idea! You can actually re-script, re-enact, and rehearse the dreams to become something favorable and memorable. You can use storyboards, visuals, or art to retell your dreams.

Defining Your Dreams

You may have a lot of aspirations that you consider dreams. Maybe you dream about a new car, a better job, a nice house, a long-term relationship, time and money to travel the world, time and money to help others, a new career, or winning the lottery. Are all of these dreams? Goals, maybe, but it's doubtful they are all dreams. How do you tell the difference? The following is a quick brainstorming exercise you can do to cull out the goals (or wants) from the dreams. Ask yourself the following questions and write down the answer as quickly as possible. Don't think about them too much. What would you do if ...

- You won $1 million?

- You had to return to college to get a 4-year degree?

- You lost your present job?

- You had a disability that prevented you from walking?

- You won $1,000 a week for life?

- You had 6 months to live?

These questions should force you to look behind what you might assume to be your dream. For example, you might assume that your dream is to have lots of money—but what do you want from that money? What do you want to do with your time? With whom do you want to spend your time?

"What you can do, or dream you can, begin it. Boldness has genius, power, and magic in it."

—Goethe

MOVING FORWARD TOWARD YOUR DREAMS

Have you ever had inventors' remorse in the hardware or homewares store upon seeing some clever invention—or remake of an old invention—that you had perhaps contemplated years before? While you may have had the idea, the person who took it to fruition had the idea as well, but for him or her it became a "dream come true." The inventor followed his or her passion and created something, while you merely thought about it and then let it go. They made the idea become the dream that became the reality for them. Just like Thomas Edison and the Wright Brothers: Imagine if they had not made their dreams come true!

That's not to say putting your dreams into action is always easy. There are many hurdles and roadblocks you have to surmount. When working in the former Soviet Union on health care projects with many of my nurse colleagues from across North America, we learned some hard lessons. When a contract needed to be signed or work needed to be done on a hospital renovation project, we were repeatedly reminded that while anything is possible, not everything is probable. The dream was to rebuild the hospital to international quality standards. It was imperative to keep the dream foremost in our thoughts while struggling with all the details that had to come together to make that dream come true. We realized our dreams through persistence and tenacity. So, be persistent and reap the benefits. By building your dream—helping your dream to come to life, no matter what it may be—you build yourself.

Some "Do's" for moving forward toward your goals are:

1. **Believe in your dream.** Make sure it's something you want and can pour your heart into.

2. **Visualize your dream.** Visualizing your dream will energize you, because you can then see how the world changes for the better and how people (including you) live a happier life because of your dream. The energy and excitement is there for you to feel.

3. **Expect a hard way ahead.** Enough said.

4. **Take one bite at a time.** Set reasonable and accomplishable goals. It's no good creating hurdles so high you will inevitably fail. Set the first goals low enough that you are sure to achieve them, and set each successive series of goals more aggressively as you gain confidence in moving toward the goal.

"You may say I'm a dreamer, but I'm not the only one."

—John Lennon

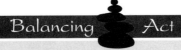

Balancing Act

DREAMING OF A FUTURE THAT COULD BE

As a young girl growing up in an abusive household, this author often dreamed of what could be. I looked at the relationships my friends had with their parents and families and wished I could have that in my life. I knew that I could be better, that I could do better, and at age 14 I set out on a mission to prove it.

"Build a dream, and the dream will build you."

—Robert Schuller

My health care career began then, at age 14, as a volunteer. At the same time, I found as many jobs as possible to generate income. The jobs were varied—from assisting an accountant with the daily receipts of a number of local food establishments to babysitting and more. I worked long hours, and I worked hard. I developed a strong work ethic from my affiliation with the accountant. He taught me the importance of completing a task in order to realize my goals. He served as a referral for me when I applied to nursing school, and he became a lifelong friend and mentor.

I knew I needed a good education to realize my dreams, and I saw nursing as the vehicle to help me achieve them. My initial program was only 3 years, leading to a diploma. I graduated with honors and went on to complete baccalaureate and master's degrees on a continuum of learning that has not yet stopped many years later.

I was fortunate to have had a role model, someone who believed in me and my ability and who helped me to understand the value of dreams.

Supporting Your Dreams?

Each and every day, people across the country and around the world are living their dreams. Are you one of them? You may think that your dreams are out of reach and impossible to achieve. But, people prove every day that someone is going to get healthy, strong, smart, rich, famous, and hopefully improve his or her life along the way.

"So many of our dreams at first seem impossible; then they seem improbable, and then, when we summon the will, they soon become inevitable."

—Christopher Reeve

Don't allow self-doubt to interfere with your success. There is no such thing as an impossible dream; only one without action steps to make it a reality. Make sure you support your dream. Share the dream and your plan with loved ones. Make sure you have people who can offer moral support on those low days.

Balancing Act

GIVE DREAMS A CHANCE

Many people experience their best dreams during the day, but the nights can yield ideas and inspiration too.

Dreams generally are associated with the sleep cycle, and it is during rapid eye movement (REM 5) sleep that we dream most deeply. One sleep cycle comprises five stages in the sleep cycle, including delta, or the first 5-10 minutes when you are falling asleep. The sleep cycle repeats itself about an average of four to five times per night, but may repeat as many as seven times. Thus, you can see how a person has several different dreams in one night. Most people, however, only remember dreams that occur closer toward the morning when they are about to wake up. But just because you can't remember those dreams does not mean that they never happened. Some people swear that they simply do not dream. In reality, they just don't remember their dreams.

Stage 1: This is known as Delta One, and we have all experienced it. Our eyes fade while driving or sitting in a classroom. This is the beginning of the sleep cycle.

Stage 2. You are entering into light sleep. This stage is characterized by non-rapid eye movements (NREM), muscle relaxation, lowered body temperature, and slowed heart rate. The body is preparing to enter into deep sleep.

Stage 3: Also characterized by NREM, this stage is defined by a further drop in body temperature and relaxation of the muscles. The body's immune system goes to work on repairing the day's damage, the endocrine glands secrete growth hormone, and blood is sent to the muscles to be reconditioned. In this stage, you are completely asleep.

Stage 4: Still in the NREM stage, this is an even deeper sleep. Your metabolic levels are extremely slow.

Stage 5: In this stage of sleep, your eyes move back and forth erratically. Referred to as REM sleep or delta sleep, this stage occurs at about 90-100 minutes after the onset of sleep. Your blood pressure rises, heart rate speeds up, respiration becomes erratic, and brain activity increases. Your involuntary muscles also become paralyzed. This stage is the most restorative part of sleep. Your mind is being revitalized and emotions are being fine tuned. The majority of your dreaming occurs in this stage.

Do you dream? Do you even sleep? A number of nurse researchers have spent their careers studying the sleep patterns of men and women. Joan Shaver, professor and dean, University of Illinois at Chicago College of Nursing, was one of the first to study sleep problems in menopausal women. Mid-afternoon tiredness may be alleviated with a glass of water; hydration is critical. Tips to fight insomnia include:

- Avoid alcohol, caffeine, and heavy, spicy or sugary foods 4-6 hours before sleep

- Stick to a daily routine

- Exercise regularly

- Block out distractions

- Practice relaxation techniques

- Establish pre-sleep rituals

- Stay hydrated, especially during afternoon periods of tiredness

Keeping Your Balance
REFLECTIONS

- What were your daydreams as a child?

- What are three dreams that you accomplished in your life? Write them down. What efforts contributed to the accomplishment of those dreams?

- What are you dreaming about doing right now that you aren't doing?

- What are the barriers to achieving your current dream? Make a list and then develop a plan for working through each one.

"It's never too late to be who you might have been."

—George Eliot (Mary Anne Evans)

10

REINVENTING YOURSELF THROUGH YOUR CAREER

Now that you've reflected on and made strides toward balancing all aspects of your life, it's time to consider *who* that rebalanced you becomes in the workplace. Has your path led you to a forked road where "straight ahead" is no longer an option? (This could be by personal choice or because the organization has changed in a way that there's no longer room for you, or your skills no longer fit the new business focus.) Or, are you merely at a crossroads where you can continue on your present course, but want to consider the options those other directions offer? Regardless of what brought you to your present place, it may be time to step back, take a deep breath, and reflect on a new vision of what a career might mean for you.

GOING FORWARD OR STEPPING BACK

Realizing you need change to get out of your rut is the first step. Once you're there, spend some time thinking about which direction you want to go. Do you want to change into a new career? Stay in the same career but move forward into a promotion? Stay in the same career but move backward into a prior job that you enjoyed, was more meaningful, and that was less stressful? Segue into an "unjob" (contract, freelance, or self-employment work) or put your career on hold (sabbatical or leave of absence) while you explore those things you always wanted to do that offer zero or minimal financial compensation? This could mean honing an art such as pottery or painting, or even exploring missionary work, nursing or spiritual.

Take the time to reflect on how your life purpose and your dreams should inform your career choices. Many of the exercises throughout the chapters can also be applied to career exploration. See "Career-Change Exercises" for some career-specific exercises. There are numerous excellent tools on the Web for career evaluation and career-change exercises and resources. One that has very good resources is Quintessential Careers (http://www.quintcareers.com/career-changer.html).

Balancing Act

CAREER CHANGE EXERCISES
By Nicholas Ricciuti: Managing Director, Everybody's Career Company

Career change can occur for a number of reasons, from the anticipated (marriage, empty nest), to the unexpected (illness, divorce, layoff), to "non-events" (a promotion that fell through, a friend got promoted, etc.).

Reflection

SWOT analysis

If you are looking for a career change to advance your own career then the SWOT (Strengths, Weaknesses, Opportunities, Threats) analysis is an excellent tool for getting an accurate and informed view of where you are right now. It should be used before making any decisions about future career choice.

The SWOT analysis shown below asks you to consider the following factors:

- What are your strengths?
- What are your weaknesses or development needs?
- What are the opportunities for development within your chosen career?
- What threats are you facing?

"Everyone thinks of changing the world, but no one thinks of changing himself."

—Leo Tolstoy

Use the following guide in thinking about the types of areas you should explore in your personal SWOT analysis. The analysis will help in clarifying career choices, such as whether to move into another role within your current organization or to exit the organization.

Strengths

List what you consider to be your most marketable skills.

How can your skills transfer to other roles in your organization, other functional areas, and other industries?

What are your best leadership qualities?

Weaknesses

What gaps in capability do you perceive you have for the role you aspire for?

What would others say are your blind spots?

How might your blind spots derail your potential?

Opportunities

What is the level of demand for the skill sets that you possess in your organization or your preferred organization?

What roles are in the planning stage for advertising?

What development strategies could you adopt to increase your chances of landing a role?

Threats

Who in the organization will be a resistance or block to your moving into this role?

What is the level of competition for this role?

Have you resigned in difficult circumstances? How will you explain this in your next interview?

You can effectively plan and manage career change through career choice analysis and the ways you choose to develop your career.

Wheel of Life—Get the Balance Right

A week consists of 168 hours. Measure and reflect over the past 3 months, and estimate the time you have spent on the following eight aspects of your life.

- **Business:** Career progression activity

- **Finance:** Investments and other monetary activities and responsibilities

- **Family:** Spouse, kids, parents, and other relatives
- **Spiritual:** Worship, community, volunteering
- **Physical:** General exercise, sports, or activity participation
- **Mental:** Reading, self-learning, formal education
- **Social:** Friends, outings, movies, having fun
- **Rest:** Sleep, "me time," relaxation, holidays

Generally, if any one of these parts of your life is taking up a lot of your time over a sustained period, other areas of your life suffer. Your career should be your passion, and contribute to your overall happiness and well-being.

Reprinted with permission from Nicholas Ricciuti, Everybody's Career Company: www.reinventyourcareer.com.au/

STAYING IN OR STARTING A NEW JOB—LIVE A PASSIONATE LIFE

Regardless of your particular career choice or situation, it is hard to maintain a level of passion about your life when those around you don't feel the same, particularly in the workplace. There are always other people who have been in dead-end jobs themselves, maybe for many years. Or, maybe some of your colleagues dislike what they do; don't have a defined purpose for being; or feel inadequate, underpaid, unloved, unappreciated, or a myriad other ways that you can probably understand yourself.

Don't let those around you drag you down, particularly when you've worked hard to balance or rebalance your life. Don't stoop to their level of unhappiness! Don't feel less passionate about what you are doing because others do not value it! Do see the opportunity to rise to the occasion and lead by example.

Rather than try to explain to others how you are feeling and what you are doing, show them with your actions. When you are joyous and productive in your daily life, others will observe that and be curious. By staying calm and cheerful, you can influence angry, noisy, and otherwise unhappy people.

"There is nothing like returning to a place that remains unchanged to find the ways in which you yourself have altered."

—Nelson Mandela

I still recall a nursing school reunion where I was the only one present without a walker, cane, or wheelchair. I knew the ages of my classmates. We had, after all, started our nursing program together at ages 17-18. My colleagues asked me what I had been doing that allowed me to be in so much better physical shape than they were. They assumed that it was some sort of miracle drug that had given me a new lease on life. Frankly, I did not need a new lease because the old one had not yet run out. My good health was my passion! And, my passion related to my newfound interest in health and wellness, as opposed to disease and sickness. I'll admit that part of this interest came with being a new grandparent and my desire to sit on the floor and play … and be able to get up again. I demonstrated, through my actions, a passion for wellness and overall well-being.

And, I remember when one of my colleagues asked if I had my knees replaced yet. I replied that the originals were still working, and I did not plan to replace them simply because I had reached a certain age. I was passionate about losing a few extra pounds that put unnecessary pressure on my knees, allowing them to last longer.

SHARE THE PASSION

Invite others to share in what you do in your life that is making such a difference. By including other people in your activities, they are more likely to be open to the changes you are experiencing in your life. People around you will respond to your efforts in showing them what you are learning and discovering.

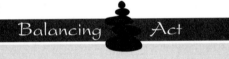

Balancing Act

FIND AND SHARE YOUR BLISS

- Set aside time for yourself every day. This can be a quiet time that you schedule into your day, every day. Use this time to think, write, read, meditate, or do anything else that will further your passions. Those around you will adjust quickly to this time and will not interrupt you. It is your time to be, and to appreciate, you.

- Focus on what you love, eliminating as much as possible what does not feed your joy or energy.

- Go with your feelings and emotions and do what feels good! So many of us have allowed others to tell us what we should do, think, and feel for so long that it might take some time for you to find your bliss. Stick with it, and the world will be at your command.

WHEN OPPORTUNITY KNOCKS, ANSWER

We are in a never-ending state of change. We are constantly growing and evolving, and it is impossible to remain the same person you are today, even if you wanted to. Think about your health care career and the number of times that you have reinvented yourself.

"In the same way as the tree bears the same fruit year after year, but each time new fruit, all lastingly valuable ideas in thinking must always be reborn."

—Albert Schweitzer

When you started out as a recent graduate, chances are that you did not immediately envision yourself as the chief nursing officer. Chances are that you thought of yourself as a clinician, or perhaps as a future educator helping to mold the minds and spirits of the next generation of future nurses. Your aspirations related to the next step or two in front of you. At some point in your clinical career, though, you chose a specialty practice and developed your skills to a level of being the best that you could be in your field—an expert. You may have become involved in leadership initiatives within your organization, maybe even become part of an elite team working on Magnet initiatives, shared governance models, or internal councils. Perhaps you joined a professional society and assumed a leadership role within that organization. If a local chapter was within your field of vision, you may have started it. If a national position was within your field of vision, perhaps you took the steps necessary and paid your dues along the way to make that a reality.

"Change is the constant, the signal for rebirth, the egg of the phoenix."
—Christina Baldwin

Don't be afraid to challenge yourself. You never know where a new experience may take you. For example, I was working in an emergency department in a community hospital before I began my infusion specialty practice. A patient arrived in acute distress and needed an intravenous infusion. I had never performed that procedure. I wasn't even trained in it. The emergency department physician challenged me to start the infusion. Back then, nurses did not learn how to start IVs. As the only nurse on duty in the ED that night, and no available supervisor, I used the resources I had available. After consulting the procedure manual and the product label, I started the infusion successfully. It was at that moment that I decided to become the best that I could be, and to learn all that I could about the practice of infusion nursing. From that moment of inspiration, I became a local and national leader, national president, director of the certification board, and eventually author of the textbook that I initially consulted for my first IV back in 1975. I reinvented myself as an infusion specialist, and I continue to evolve in my career today.

AGE IS NO OBSTACLE

It is never too late to reinvent your life, no matter how early or late it is in your career. You can do anything you want to do at any time. We all know there is an abundance of resources for those just out of school, but did you know that there's a movement for established career types called the *Third Age*? The Third Age is a life stage created by an extended life expectancy into the 80s and beyond—a time that represents new possibilities for living in fulfillment and purpose. Third agers are typically anywhere between 45 and 65, have raised their children, and face many healthy, productive years left in their lives. These are people who may need to move out of a physically demanding job—such as bedside nursing—but plan to work for a number of years before retiring, or they may be retirees who need to—or choose to—return to work for income, personal enrichment, or social reasons.

"Human beings have an inalienable right to invent themselves."

—Germaine Greer

Many people may feel that they are too old and lack enough education, money, or time to do what they really want to do. But that is not true. What *is* true is what, in your mind's eye, you see as possible. Look at where you are now and move toward that which you want to become. AARP (formerly the American Association of Retired Persons) offers wonderful resources for those third agers considering a career change or looking for a new job (http://www.aarp.org/money/work).

LIVE AN INTENTIONAL LIFE

As you continue to find balance, remember that whatever opportunities appear in your life, you are equipped to handle

139

them and handle them well. Full participation on an emotional, physical, spiritual, and intellectual level enhances your life and that of those around you. Keep an open mind—open to other areas of life to which you may not have been exposed. Create a calendar of places to go and people to see. This might include something you have been longing to do, or something that you perhaps thought about, but never dared to do.

A colleague recently took a job in a retail store because she plans to open her own retail business by the end of the year. Although she is working in ladies wear, the customer service model is similar to her own vision of a business. She has already applied through the Small Business Administration for funding, and she wants to open her restaurant and tea café close to home and enjoy the camaraderie of a steady stream of "regulars." I met her at a networking event through the local Chamber of Commerce, and initially thought of her as a business colleague. By actively listening to her, I realized that she was a certified hematology/oncology nurse who lost her passion for nursing, but not for people, so she's reinventing herself.

I thought of my nursing school roommate. A diploma graduate, she went on to obtain a baccalaureate degree from the University of Pennsylvania and became a master's prepared neonatal nurse specialist. Years later, as she traveled with her physician husband to new assignments, she also lost her passion for nursing, but not for people. She opened an antique shop in a small town and has enjoyed tremendous success.

"Each decision we make, each action we take, is born out of an intention."
—Sharon Salzberg

Sometimes our identity gets lost or buried over the years, and we realize we have not done the things that we always dreamed of doing, such as traveling, starting our own wellness business, opening an antique shop, or building a community around a tea café. It is important to visualize those things by writing them down and revisiting the thoughts that you left behind.

Balancing Act

DOWN MEMORY LANE

You have the power to reinvent yourself at any point in your life. Age, position, job, circumstances: None of these should stand in your way. Think about how quickly Thanksgiving dinner turns into conversations that begin, "Hey, remember when we ..." We recall some events imperfectly, and others may not have occurred or are remembered differently by other people. But, it remains great fun to share the stories as well as the memories. It is like a walk down memory lane. In a personal development program, I participated in a game called "Down Memory Lane." The concept was to remember yourself as a small child, and to think about what brought you satisfaction in life, what may have frightened you, and your responses.

Take time to walk down memory lane. Write down what brought you great satisfaction—that is what you want to focus on as you move forward in life. Write down what brought you least satisfaction—avoid those as much as possible!

"Change is not merely necessary to life—it is life."

—Alvin Toffler

AFFIRMATIONS

You have a full caseload, a full workweek, family responsibilities, and more! You have the power within to change lives each and every day of your career. A staff nurse on an inpatient psychiatric unit understands how behavioral health disorders interfere with the ability to interact with others in a life-affirming way. We all need interaction and affirmation in our lives. I have made a daily habit of stating and repeating affirmations aloud that support my passion for being. For example, I might say, "Today someone, somewhere will benefit from my act of kindness."

What about you? As a nursing professional, your own priorities are usually not about you. When, as a nursing professional, do you have time to debrief? When, as a nursing professional, do you take the time to encourage others to pursue a nursing career? Think about and identify your core values; prioritize your needs; and then dream the big dream. Is this the right time to reinvent yourself and your nursing career? Think of those who have done it successfully and be willing to know the real you! You can do it, as no one else can.

Keeping Your Balance

PRACTICE A DAILY PLAN FOR REINVENTION

Every day is a new beginning and an opportunity to reinvent oneself. Begin with 10-20 minutes of meditation or quiet time. Picture yourself living the life of your dreams. This can be difficult sometimes, because we are so caught up with the reality of our daily lives. But don't let reality get in the way of your dreams. Whatever you think about and picture in your mind's eye, you are capable of manifesting into your life.

We are indeed spiritual beings living a physical experience, not the other way around. Expect miracles from your life every day. Remember that everything in our material world was once someone's abstract dream. If we did not dream for the future, we would not have the things that we give so much value to today.

"I seldom end up where I wanted to go, but almost always end up where I need to be."

—Douglas Adams

11

DESTINY IN THE BALANCE

We all assume many roles in life—our roles in the family, in the workplace, in our physical community, and in our professional community. Each role allows us to express a different dimension of our being. It is these separate roles that need to be balanced in our lives. For example, your life needs balancing if you are professionally successful, but family members complain that you do not spend enough time with them. Your lifestyle needs balancing if, again, your career is soaring but your health is challenged. Finally, if you are addicted to a favorite TV show but have no time to clean your closets or the garage—your life needs balancing.

"Gather only what you need; travel lightly, and keep moving forward. The journey will be more joyful with less baggage."

—Deborah Haggerty

ATTITUDE

Your destiny lies in achieving balance, and there are two major ways in which to balance your life. Since life coexists with time, the first way to balance life is to balance time. Many outstanding publications address time management, some of which are specific to nursing professionals. Find the ones that suit your style and needs, and use them! The second way to balance life is by balancing one's attitude—the secret word is *attitude*. Attitude is critical to success in life. Some call it a winning or a positive attitude. Everything flows from it. Basically, things work best for those who make the best of the way things work out.

Many years ago, a large American shoe manufacturer sent two sales representatives to different parts of the Australian outback to see if they could generate business among the aborigine people. Some time later, the company received messages from both agents. The first one said, "No business here; natives don't wear shoes." The second one said, "Great opportunity here; natives don't wear shoes." If you can't change your fate—if you can't see a market for shoes among people who don't wear them—change your attitude.

"Nothing can stop the man with the right mental attitude from achieving his goal; nothing on earth can help the man with the wrong mental attitude."

—Thomas Jefferson

While we all would like to be successful, many have reasons upon reasons why they cannot succeed. In truth, all we need is one reason why we *can*. That reason is attitude. Nothing is more important—not education, aptitude, health, wealth, or opportunity.

What, then, is attitude? Attitude is our disposition, perspective, viewpoint, or outlook. It is how we view the world. If we perceive the glass as half-full, it is; if we perceive it as half-empty, it is. That is, we don't see things as they are; we see things as we are—we interpret our experiences, labeling them as good or bad. However, our interpretations do not affect reality; they just affect us.

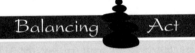

Balancing Act

SMILE THERAPY

It may seem or feel silly at first, but challenge yourself to smile at everyone you meet for one full day. Don't worry if they don't smile back. Just keep smiling. By the end of the day, you'll be happier, as smiling creates energy while frowning takes energy.

"The greatest discovery of my generation is that human beings can alter their lives by altering their attitudes of mind."

—William James

Some people, for instance, love cold weather; others hate it. Obviously, our feelings have no influence on the temperature, as no matter how angry or grumpy we get about the cold temperature, it won't get warmer.

Our emotions have great impact on our lives, bringing us happiness or unhappiness. Some of us can discover opportunity in every difficulty; others find nothing but difficulty in every opportunity—same circumstances, but different perspective, thus different attitudes.

One way to change your life is to change your attitude. "How?" you may ask. It's simple, really; just behave the way you want to become. Are you a pessimist that wishes to become an optimist? If so, pretend to be optimistic. When you change your behavior, you change everything within your worldview. At first, it might feel forced, but the longer you do it, the more it becomes a habit—a positive habit—that will be just as easy to live in as your old pessimistic patterns. The world is a mirror, so behave as if you are happy. When you do that, the world will reflect back happiness. Be downcast, and the world responds similarly. It is not the position, but the *disposition* that makes this possible.

"We who lived in concentration camps can remember the men who walked through the huts comforting others, giving away their last piece of bread. They may have been few in number, but they offer sufficient proof that everything can be taken from a man but one thing: the last of the human freedoms— to choose one's attitude in any given set of circumstances, to choose one's own way."

—Victor Frankl

THE POWER OF POSITIVE THINKING

- Use positive action words when talking and thinking. Phrases such as "I can" and "I will" are powerful and help support attitude change. Carry this through into all your conversations.

- Push out all feelings that aren't positive. Don't let negative thoughts and feelings overwhelm you when you're feeling down. Even if it's only for a few hours a day, push your negativity aside and only focus on the good things in your life.

- Surround yourself with positive people.

- Before starting with any plan or action, visualize clearly in your mind its successful outcome. If you visualize with concentration and faith, you will be amazed at the results.

- Always sit and walk with your back straight. This will strengthen your confidence and inner strength.

FIVE PILLARS OF LIFE

Let's re-examine the five pillars of life that impact our balance and destiny. We advance in life by setting goals, and these goals are specific to mind, body, family, society, and career/finances.

1. **MIND** is the first pillar. A healthy mind is tantamount to success.

2. **BODY** is next. A healthy body is obtained through exercise, a proper diet, and quality sleep.

3. **FAMILY** provides us with the chance to express love and assume and share responsibility.

4. **SOCIETY** is an opportunity to give back, to pay it forward, and to tap into a power greater than ourselves. An appreciation of morality, the arts, wonder, awe, and nature will heighten our awareness of the spiritual dimension.

5. **CAREER** (finances) is our opportunity to earn income to provide our essential needs, express ourselves, mentor others, and develop our personal and professional growth.

"What we see depends mainly on what we look for."

—Sir John Lubbock

Balancing Act

FINDING THE FIVE PILLARS

With the Five Pillars of Life in mind, ask yourself these questions:

- Which two of these five pillars are most important to me? Why are they important?

- Which two of these are most out of balance for me? What would it take to bring them into balance?

- What would I be willing to do to have these things in my life?

- What would I be willing to give up?

- Do I believe this is possible for me?

"While the fates permit, live happily; life speeds on with hurried step, and with winged days the wheel of the headlong year is turned."

—Seneca

Remember, we are all unique. It is unreasonable to expect everyone to perfectly balance each role in life. Further, there will be times in our lives where we focus more on one aspect of our lives than another. The important lesson is not about balancing our lives perfectly, but about balancing them in a manner that best expresses our potential and that gives us the most health and joy. We do this by adhering to the rule of *BE...DO...HAVE.*

You have to *BE* self-disciplined to *DO* what is needed to balance your life; when you do so, you will *HAVE* balance in the five pillars.

CHANGE BEGINS WITH CHOICE

Any day we wish, we can discipline ourselves to change it all. Any day we wish, we can open the book that will open our mind to new knowledge. Any day we wish, we can start a new activity. Any day we wish, we can start the process of life change. We can do it immediately, next week, next month, or next year. We can also do nothing, but you wouldn't be reading this book if that was a choice you were looking for.

"Destiny is no matter of chance. It is a matter of choice. It is not a thing to be waited for, it is a thing to be achieved."

—William Jennings

Consider the following as you reinvent yourself:

1. **Keep your options open.** Don't turn down opportunities just because they are outside the parameters of what you have thought to be your job title or place in life. The real opportunity might be behind a previously closed door.

2. **Cross-pollinate.** Take your knowledge, skills, and abilities from one field to another. Step outside your comfort zone. Look for ideas to bring into your field from others. Plant your ideas within entirely new fields, new pastures.

3. **Follow your heart's desire and live your passion.** Your heart is a wise barometer of what you need to be doing with your life. Think from the heart as well as the mind when you evaluate opportunities. Don't live by the dreams of others. Rather, live your own dreams.

4. **Live a little.** If you went to graduate school right out of university without taking time to experience life, do it now. Experience often prods us to do something beyond our wildest imaginations. The more experiences you accumulate, the more you get a view of what works for you and what doesn't. These experiences provide the basis for ongoing reinventions of self.

5. **Visualize.** Paint a picture in your mind's eye of what you want in your life. I often print out the words, attach a photo, and hang it on my bulletin board. It is what I see in the morning when I enter my office, and what I see later in the day. It is a constant reminder of what I expect to achieve and what I believe is within my reach. Take every chance to experience this inner image with all of your five senses.

6. **Be curious.** Keep your eyes and ears open and your antenna up for new people and new ideas to enter your life. You have heard that it is not what you know, but who you know that counts. This has never been truer than in the field of reinvention.

7. **Network with like-minded people.** Make a point to meet new people as often as you can. New people in your life will enrich you and lead you to new opportunities. Don't make it about you; listen actively to what others say in the networking community. Be a giver, because givers gain.

"No trumpets sound when the important decisions of our life are made. Destiny is made known silently."

—Agnes de Mille

At some point in your life, you have to make a decision. You have to change. Change is a constant, an essential catalyst for reinventing ourselves, our lives, and our work. Change usually takes courage and tenacity, especially when there is no guarantee of success. Change is a process of reinvention.

OUT OF THE MOUTHS OF BABES

In his book *Career Reexplosion: Reinvent Yourself in Thirty Days,* Gary Joseph Grappo suggests that changing your career can change your life. To arrive at three new career directions to explore, he suggests this simple exercise:

- List at least 10 childhood experiences, situations, events, hobbies, interests, skills, education, and so on that you enjoyed and made you happy.

- Repeat this list for activities that have made you happy throughout your adult years.

- Place these lists side by side and list your top 10 dream careers that may be derived from the dreams, passions, and experiences you have accumulated from the two lists. Brainstorm with those you respect most, conduct an Internet search, and create the career of your vision and dreams without worrying about the education, money, or resources you'd need to achieve them.

- Narrow your wish list down to the top three reinvention choices, keeping in mind they will be fluid and subject to change. Then, take action toward them and watch what happens. Reinvention is about a decision, a commitment, and action steps in support of that decision. Make the decision yours and yours alone.

BALANCING WITH THE BEST OF THEM

The core of a balanced life is congruence with your values, dreams, and goals. How your life balances is up to you. You are the driver of your own bus! Once you have determined where you are out of balance and how to rebalance, you will be primed to succeed like never before. Make a positive attitude an integral part of everything you do, and you will succeed faster than you ever imagined.

"Bless not only the road but the bumps on the road. They are all part of the higher journey."

—Julia Cameron

Keeping Your Balance

PILLARS OF GOOD HEALTH

This final exercise helps you get ready to apply the principles you have learned in all aspects of your daily lives.

Write what you want to be, do, or have in each of the following categories:

HEALTHY BODY

HEALTHY MIND

HEALTHY FAMILY

HEALTHY SOCIETY

HEALTHY WORKPLACE

Now develop a plan to achieve your goals. Be sure to take small steps. For example, start with just one small goal in one area, and let success build your confidence as you move from one area to the next.

REFERENCES

CHAPTER 1

Alderfer, C. (1972). *Existence, relatedness, and growth: Human needs in organizational settings.* New York: Free Press.

Associated Press. (2007, August 21). *Poll: 1 in 4 U.S. adults read no books last year.* Retrieved December 17, 2008, from http://www.iht.com/articles/ap/2007/08/21/america/NA-GEN-US-Reading-Habits-AP-Poll.php

Frankl, V. (1977). *Man's search for meaning.* New York: Pocket Books.

Friedman, T. (2005). *The world is flat: A brief history of the twenty-first century.* New York: Farrar, Straus & Giroux.

Maslow, A.H. (1943). A theory of human motivation. *Psychological Review, 50*(4), 370-396.

CHAPTER 2

Davidson, R.J., Kabat-Zinn, J., Schumacher, J., Rosenkranz, M., Muller, D., Santorelli, S.F., et al. (2003). Alterations in brain and immune function produced by mindfulness meditation. *Psychosomatic Medicine, 65*(4), 564-570.

CHAPTER 3

Naska, A., Oikoniomou, E., Trichopoulou, A., Psaltopoulou, T., & Trichopoulos, D. (2007). Siesta in healthy adults and coronary mortality in the general population. *Archives in Internal Medicine, 167*(3), 296-301.

NIOSH. (n.d.). *Stress at work.* NIOSH Publication No. 99-101. Retrieved October 8, 2008, from http://www.cdc.gov/niosh/stresswk.html

Sarnataro, B.R. (n.d.). *Top 10 fitness facts: Some things you should know about exercise.* Retrieved October 8, 2008, from http://www.webmd.com/fitness-exercise/guide/exercise-benefits

Scott, E. (2008). *Sleep benefits: Power napping for increased productivity, stress relief, and health.* Retrieved October 8, 2008, from http://stress.about.com/od/lowstresslifestyle/a/powernap.htm

Steptoe, A., & Brydon, L. (2005). Association between acute lipid stress responses and fasting lipid levels 3 years later. *Health Psychology, 24*(6), 601-607.

CHAPTER 4

Pagana, K.P. (2008). *The nurse's etiquette advantage: How professional etiquette can advance your nursing career.* Indianapolis, IN: Sigma Theta Tau International.

CHAPTER 5

Navarro, D. (2006). *How to stay focused. Rock your day: Stop settling for less, start changing your life.* Retrieved December 8, 2008, from http://www.rockyourday.com/how-to-stay-focused/

CHAPTER 6

Ardell, D.B. (1986). *High level wellness* (10th ed.). Berkeley, CA: Ten Speed Press.

Careerbuilder. (2006, May 3). *Three out of four workers report burnout on the job, CareerBuilder.com survey finds.* Retrieved December 8, 2008, from http://www.careerbuilder.com/share/aboutus/pressreleasesdetail.aspx?id=pr303&sd=5%2f3%2f2006&ed=12%2f31%2f2006&siteid=cbprCBPR303&sc_cmp1=cb_pr303_

Covey, S. (2004). *The 7 habits of highly effective people.* Florence, MA: Free Press.

Harris Interactive. (2005). *The Harris Poll #38. Many U.S. employees have negative attitudes to their jobs, employers, and top managers.* Retrieved December 8, 2008, from http://www.harrisinteractive.com/harris_poll/index.asp?PID=568

Littell, B. (n.d.). *Part 1 – Introduction to NetWeaving.* Retrieved January 8, 2009, from http://www.netweaving.com/articles/ Part1-IntrotoNWing.pdf

Nash, L., & Stevenson, H. (2004). *Just enough: Tools for creating success in your work and life.* New York: John Wiley.

CHAPTER 7

American Nurses Association. (2008). *2008 ANA house of delegates healthy food in health care action report.* Retrieved January 13, 2009, from http://www.bioscienceresource.org/documents/ ANAOppositionPolicytorBGH-June2008.pdf

Centers for Disease Control. (n.d.). *Concentrated animal feeding operations (CAFOs).* Retrieved December 16, 2008, from http://www.cdc. gov/cafos/about.htm

C.S. Mott Children's Hospital, the University of Michigan Department of Pediatrics and Communicable Diseases, and the University of Michigan Child Health Evaluation and Research. (2007, May 2). *National poll on children's health.* Retrieved December 19, 2008, from http://www.med.umich.edu/mott/research/ chearhealthconcernpoll.html

Health Care Without Harm. (n.d.). *Position statement on rBGH.* Retrieved January 13, 2009, from http://www.noharm.org/ details.cfm?ID=1104&type=document

Kirshenbaum, M. (2003). *Emotional energy factor: The secrets high-energy people use to beat emotional fatigue.* New York: Delacorte Press.

Oregon Physicians for Social Responsibility. (2003). *Know your milk: Does it have artificial hormones?* Retrieved January 13, 2009, from http://www.psr.org/site/DocServer/Brochure2007_Final. pdf?docID=4521

Union of Concerned Scientists. (2006). *They eat what? The reality of feed at animal factories.* Retrieved December 16, 2008, from http:// www.ucsusa.org/food_and_agriculture/science_and_impacts/ impacts_industrial_agriculture/they-eat-what-the-reality-of.html

CHAPTER 8

American Holistic Nurses Association. (1997). *Core curriculum for holistic nursing.* New York: Aspen Publishers.

Berk, L.S., Tan, S.A., Fry, W.F., Napier, B.J., Lee, J.W., Hubbard, R.W., et al. (1989). Neuroendocrine and stress hormone changes during mirthful laughter. *American Journal of the Medical Sciences, 298*(6), 390-396.

Bachorowski, J. (2001). Not all laughs are alike: Voiced but not unvoiced laughter readily elicits positive affect. *Psychological Science, 12*(3), 252–257.

Cousins, N. (1979). *Anatomy of an illness as perceived by the patient.* New York: Norton.

Doskoch, P. (1996, July/August). Happily ever laughter: Is humor the forgotten key to happiness? *Psychology Today.* Retrieved December 9, 2008, from http://www.psychologytoday.com/articles/pto-19960701-000032.html

Hayashi, T., Urayama-O, K.K., Hayashi, K., Iwanaga, S., Ohta, M., Saito, T., et al. (2006). Laughter regulates gene expression in patients with type 2 diabetes. *Psychotherapy and Psychosomatics, 75*(1), 62-65.

Matsuzaki, T., Nakajima, A., Ishigami, S., Tanno, M., & Yoshion, S. (2006). Mirthful laughter differentially affects serum pro- and anti-inflammatory cytokine levels depending on the level of disease activity in patients with rheumatoid arthritis. *Rheumatology, 45*(2), 182-186.

Miller, M. (2000, November/December). *Laughter is good for your heart, according to a new University of Maryland Medical Center study.* Retrieved November 15, 2008, from http://www.umm.edu/news/releases/laughter.htm

Provine, R. (2000, November/December). The science of laughter. *Psychology Today.* Retrieved January 13, 2009, from http://www.psychologytoday.com/articles/pto-20001101-000036.html

Provine, R. (2004). Laughing, tickling, and the evolution of speech and self. *Current Directions in Psychological Science, 13*(6), 215-218.

CHAPTER 11

Grappo, G. (2000). *Career reexplosion: Reinvent yourself in 30 days.* New York: Putnam.

Johnson, S. (1998). *Who moved my cheese?* New York: Penguin Group.

APPENDIX
TWENTY-SIX PRINCIPLES OF LIFE

One way to achieve balance is by living out the following 26 principles of life that enhance our overall being. These principles are reprinted with the permission of Jason Johns from turtlebowbear.com.

1. **All Are Related:** A Native American saying translates roughly to *all are related*. Everything in the universe is part of The Great Spirit, from rock to plant to fish to humans. The spirit flows between and within us all and is the building block of everything. Since we are all part of the same whole, we should treat the rest of the whole as if it were part of us: with compassion and love. We are all part of the Great Spirit, just like all the different leaves on a tree are still part of the whole tree.

2. **The Energy Flow:** The universe is composed of energy, and it flows between everything and within us all. When we have internal blocks, the energy fails to flow correctly, causing illness, lethargy, and other symptoms of dis-ease. This energy can be directed consciously; we can see it and feel it. How we feel affects our energy levels—negativity drains energy; positivity creates energy.

3. **We Are Beings of Both Spirit and Flesh:** We are spirits as well as creatures of the flesh. We inhabit both worlds simultaneously, even though we are often unaware of it. We walk with one foot in each of these worlds and must pay attention to them both. Neglecting either world causes distress in the other.

4. **No One Entity Is Superior to Another:** No one being or creature is any greater or lesser than another. We are all the same and although we are on different paths and have different levels of understanding, these differences do not make any one of us better than another. Humans are masters neither of nature, nor of animals and plants. They are our companions and co-inhabitants of this planet. We are not superior to them, nor do we own them. Treat all with respect.

5. **Belief Creates:** Our perceptions of the universe are based on our beliefs. If we believe we are in a hurry, then everyone else appears to be going slow. Through belief and positive thought, we can create virtually anything. Believe in our abilities and ourselves, and we will succeed. We can combine the power of belief with that of visualization to bring anything into reality.

6. **Intuition:** Inside of us, a voice—intuition—speaks and guides us. We can choose to ignore or listen to it. Once we are in tune with our intuition and start to

listen to it, we will be guided and will find that we can achieve more than we thought possible. We will begin to realize that the Great Spirit works through us—often in mysterious ways, but always to our benefit—over the long term.

7. **The Higher Purpose:** Everything that happens is for a reason and for the greater good. Learn to look at events in our lives from more than just the accepted human perspective. We must see them from the perspective of the Great Spirit and contemplate what good will come from these events. This is the old maxim of, "Is the glass half full or half empty?" We can look at events negatively, as half empty, or positively, as half full. A positive or optimistic view creates more energy and helps us act more effectively.

8. **There Are No Ordinary Moments:** The past only exists in our memory. The future only exists as our expectation. The now is what really matters most. It is a precious moment and it is important that we treat every single moment as special and live it to its fullest. By being in the present, we have presence. To live in the "now" the conscious mind should be quiet: Focus totally on what you are doing, not what you are going to be doing in the future.

9. **There Are No Limits:** The only limits we have are those we place upon our abilities and potentials. To this end, do not accept being labeled by others. If someone views a dog as being vicious, then it is more likely to be vicious. Hold no expectations of others and let them be themselves, just as we would be ourselves.

10. **Action Not Reaction:** If we are tickled, our reaction is to laugh. Consciously develop a state of

awareness where we can act, rather than react, in any situation. Reaction is unconscious, whereas action is conscious. Do not let past influences affect your present actions. For example, if you were once bitten by a dog, do not act fearful around the next dog you meet, expecting that it will also bite. There are times to act, as well as times to be still. By living in the present and having control of the conscious mind, we can better direct our action.

11. **Positivity Rules:** Negative thoughts attract negative events and drain our energy. Surround yourself with positive people and positivity will come your way. Positive thoughts attract positive events and increase our energy. To this end, it is most helpful to look at our thoughts and the events that happen to us in a positive light and release negative thoughts.

12. **Posture, Pose, and Breathing:** Energy flows through the body, as it flows through all things. If the posture and pose are bad, the energy cannot flow cleanly and becomes blocked, which manifests as pain or illness. We breathe in energy from the world around us. Therefore, our breaths should be deep and full, coming from the bottom of the belly and not the chest or shoulders. This enables us to maximize our energy. Deep breathing helps relax us. When we are stressed, angry, or afraid, our breathing changes and becomes shallow and faster. By consciously controlling our breathing and keeping it deep and even, we can release stress, anger, or fear, enabling us to act consciously in the situation.

13. **Everything in Balance:** The universe exists in a state of balance, as should we. We can do anything we wish, but doing it in moderation, never to excess,

promotes balance. When we do things to excess, they
can become addictive, drain energy, and may become
negative. Being balanced allows us to act better in situations. If we are sitting on the fence, so to speak, we can
jump off either way we desire or not at all.

14. **Intent Is Action:** You can intend to do anything, and
your intent is important. However, unless the intent is
followed with action, then the intent is nothing. As an
example, I may intend to get fit, but spend all my time
sitting in front of the TV eating pizza and drinking
cola. I have my intention, but my actions do not confirm or create the intention. Therefore, if you intend
to do something, do it, don't just talk about it. Action
turns knowledge into wisdom.

15. **Freedom of Choice:** We all have free will and can
choose to do anything we wish. There is no situation
where we do not have choice. It may appear that we do
not, but there are always options—if we have the pa-
tience and strength to take them. We just have to have
the courage of conviction to make the decisions.

16. **Change Happens:** Through change we can grow and
go forward. Change is continuous and is always hap-
pening around us. The simple story of *Who Moved My
Cheese?* by Spencer Johnson reveals profound truths
about change that give people and organizations a
quick and easy way to successfully change. The parable
enables readers to recognize change, prepare for it, and
deal with it. (http://www.whomovedmycheese.com)

17. **Taking Responsibility:** Our actions cause reactions—
this is a law of nature. We have to be aware of our actions and take responsibility for the consequences of
our actions. By taking responsibility for our actions, we
can take back our power and freedom to choose. We

have to accept that no one will live for us, and that sometimes our actions will cause others, or ourselves, a measure of discomfort. Remember, though, that discomfort is one way of helping us grow and showing us where changes need to be made.

18. **One Step at a Time:** Goal setting is tantamount to success. Well-conceived goals are accompanied by action plans aimed at completion. To achieve any goal, break it down into a number of small steps. Many small successes will lead to a big success. Remember that a journey toward any destination starts with a single step, then a second, a third, and as many as required until you reach your destination. Remember to reward and praise yourself for your successes, however small. By acknowledging them, you increase your power and will to succeed, strengthening your belief in yourself.

19. **Judgment:** We have no right to judge others for their words, thoughts, or deeds. They have the freedom of choice to do as they please and act as they wish, just as we do. We are in no position to judge anyone, as we are imperfect ourselves. By having no preconceptions of other people, we can interact better with them and perhaps make a new friend.

20. **Integrity:** Integrity is all about how we act when no one is looking. We must live according to our own standards and not judge others by them. This is about living in line with our highest vision despite urges to the contrary.

21. **Air Your Doubts:** Airing your doubts, fears, and worries allows you to see them for what they are, making it more likely you can conquer and release

them, ridding yourself of their burden. Refusing to confront them, however, allows them to gain power over you and become even more deeply rooted.

22. **Failure:** Failure is not something to be feared or worried over, because we can never fail! Everything we do, no matter whether we view it as a success or failure, is a valuable lesson for us to learn. By looking at a perceived failure as a valuable lesson, it no longer feels as bad. The only true failure is not learning from our mistakes.

23. **The Ongoing Journey:** Our journey of exploration through life never stops. The destination is not the reward or the goal. Rather, the journey to the destination is the goal.

24. **Don't Mind:** If we take an objective view of our mind, then we can see that lots of thoughts drift through it, many of which we are unaware. A sad, angry, or fearful thought may drift up from the subconscious and change how we feel for no apparent reason. We must take control of the mind through tools such as meditation, so we become aware of these thoughts and see them for what they are. Then, we can let them go and stay relaxed and centered. Consciously focusing on our breathing, keeping it deep and even, helps us to release these negative thoughts.

25. **Emotions:** Emotions come and go. They flow through us all the time, often without our even realizing it. Many of us do not express our emotions due to fear of what others may think or how they might respond. Emotions are to be celebrated and expressed.

26. **Play:** Remember to play, to have fun, to express joy in living. As children, we play exuberantly. We have fun, enjoy ourselves, and have lots of energy. Then something happens. We grow up and no longer play, believing that adults have to be "grown up" and not play. Playing is one of our greatest sources of pleasure. It takes many forms, from athletic sport to games, to laughing and joking with friends. Playing increases our energy and makes us more positive. It makes those around us more positive and generally lifts the spirits of all involved.

INDEX

T

U-V-W

X-Y-Z

BOOKS PUBLISHED BY THE
HONOR SOCIETY OF NURSING,
SIGMA THETA TAU INTERNATIONAL

B Is for Balance: A Nurse's Guide for Enjoying Life at Work and at Home, Weinstein, 2008.

Ready, Set, Go Lead! A Primer for Emerging Health Care Leaders, Dickenson-Hazard, 2008.

Words of Wisdom From Pivotal Nurse Leaders, Houser and Player, 2008.

Tales From The Pager Chronicles, Rancour, 2008.

The Nurse's Etiquette Advantage, Pagana, 2008.

NURSE: A World of Care, Jaret, 2008. Published by Emory University and distributed by the Honor Society of Nursing, Sigma Theta Tau International.

Nursing Without Borders: Values, Wisdom, Success Markers, Weinstein and Brooks, 2007.

Synergy: The Unique Relationship Between Nurses and Patients, Curley, 2007.

Conversations With Leaders: Frank Talk From Nurses (and Others) on the Front Lines of Leadership, Hansen-Turton, Sherman, and Ferguson, 2007.

Pivotal Moments in Nursing: Leaders Who Changed the Path of a Profession, Houser and Player, 2004 (Volume I) and 2007 (Volume II).

Daily Miracles: Stories and Practices of Humanity and Excellence in Health Care, Briskin and Boller, 2006.

A Daybook for Nurse Leaders and Mentors. Sigma Theta Tau International, 2006.

The HeART of Nursing: Expressions of Creative Art in Nursing, Second Edition, Wendler, 2005.

Making a Difference: Stories from the Point of Care, volumes I & II, Hudacek, 2005.

A Daybook for Nurses: Making a Difference Each Day, Hudacek, 2004.

Ordinary People, Extraordinary Lives: The Stories of Nurses, Smeltzer and Vlasses, 2003.

For more information and to order these books from the Honor Society of Nursing, Sigma Theta Tau International, visit the society's Web site at www.nursingsociety.org/publications, or go to www.nursingknowledge.org/stti/books, the Web site of Nursing Knowledge International, the honor society's sales and distribution division. Or, call 1.888.NKI.4.YOU (U.S. and Canada) or +1.317.634.8171 (Outside U.S. and Canada).